The Burnout Doctor

Dr Claire Ashley

The Burnout Doctor

Your 6-Step Recovery Plan

GREEN TREE

GREEN TREE
Bloomsbury Publishing Plc
50 Bedford Square, London, WC1B 3DP, UK
29 Earlsfort Terrace, Dublin 2, Ireland

BLOOMSBURY, GREEN TREE and the Green Tree logo are trademarks of Bloomsbury Publishing Plc

First published in Great Britain 2025

Bloomsbury Publishing Plc does not have any control over, or responsibility for, any third-party websites referred to or in this book. All internet addresses given in this book were correct at the time of going to press. The author and publisher regret any inconvenience caused if addresses have changed or sites have ceased to exist, but can accept no responsibility for any such changes.

Disclaimer: The material contained in this book is for informational purposes only. No material in this publication is intended to be a substitute for professional medical advice, diagnosis or treatment. Always seek the advice of your GP or other qualified health care professional with any questions you may have regarding a medical condition, including mental health concerns, or treatment and before undertaking a new healthcare regime, and never disregard professional medical advice or delay in seeking it because of something you have read in this book.

A catalogue record for this book is available from the British Library.

Library of Congress Cataloguing-in-Publication data has been applied for.

ISBN: TPB: 978-1-3994-1280-3; eBook: 978-1-3994-1278-0

2 4 6 8 10 9 7 5 3 1

Typeset in IBM Plex Serif by Deanta Global Publishing Services, Chennai, India
Printed and bound in Great Britain by CPI Group (UK) Ltd, Croydon CR0 4YY

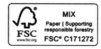

To find out more about our authors and books visit www.bloomsbury.com
and sign up for our newsletters

Contents

Introduction

None of us expect our jobs to actively harm us, but that is exactly what mine did to me. I am a practising doctor with a degree in neuroscience and I have over 20 years of medical training and clinical experience under my belt. However, despite this, even I didn't recognise that I was sliding into burnout until I hit a mental health crisis.

I'm not the only one. According to a 2024 report, a whopping 91 per cent of adults in the UK have experienced high or extreme levels of pressure and stress at some point in the past year. So, if you are feeling increasingly stressed and overwhelmed from your work or caring commitments, I hear you. I've been there. I know what it feels like. And I'm here to help you do something about it. There *is* a way through.

My own experience with burnout began just six short months after qualifying as a GP (general practitioner or family physician) – this was all the time it took for me to go from never having had a mental health problem to being in complete crisis mode. The changes that happened to my mind and body as a result of my burnout were so significant that every aspect of my life was affected and I didn't recognise the person I'd become. I can't put into words how devastating it was to experience a full-blown burnout. I wouldn't wish it on anyone, and that's exactly why I'm writing this book.

You see, despite burnout affecting so many of us today, there is still so little information readily available to support those of us who experience the condition. As an experienced doctor with a background in neuroscience, 'burnout' was not a term I had *ever* come across before – either professionally or as part of any of my training – until I had my own first-hand experience with it.

This is why I have chosen to dedicate my career to burnout education, mental health advocacy and career coaching, and why you're reading this now. There is more that can be done and more information to share, and I am here to help. During this guide I will bring together my 20-plus years of clinical training and practice, my background in neuroscience and my lived experience of burnout to help explain everything you need to know to both effectively prevent and recover from burnout. You'll have the tools, techniques and knowledge that I wish I'd had to help me.

Who can this book help?

I appreciate that the reasons why you may have picked up this book will probably vary.

Perhaps you work in a stressful job and are wondering if you're currently burned out, or perhaps you feel like you're headed there. Maybe you know that you are run down and burned out already and you need support. You might have experienced burnout and are now going through the recovery process. It could also be that you're worried about someone else and are looking for ways to understand their situation and support them. Regardless of your reasons for picking up this book, I'm glad that you have because I'm confident that this guide will give you the valuable insights and strategies to help you with your particular needs.

So, to clarify, this book is for you if you:

- work in a high-stress, high-demand job;
- often feel exhausted and overwhelmed;
- feel that you are not supported emotionally in your job, or that the demands of your job outstrip your current resources or capacity;
- are worried that your ability to manage work stress is getting away from you;

- are a woman or a member of a marginalised group, or a parent or caregiver, alongside having a high-stress job;
- identify as being burned out, but are not sure what you need to do next in order to start to recover effectively;
- are in burnout recovery, looking for guidance about what changes to make to ensure a successful, sustained recovery;
- are worried that someone close to you might be burned out.

What will we cover?

The successful management of burnout is – unfortunately – so much more than some simple self-care and stress-reduction strategies. I'll be working here, therefore, to upskill you with everything you need to know about burnout management.

My hope is that the information I provide will support some of you in preventing burnout (as, interestingly, the advice given for prevention of burnout is almost exactly the same advice as is given for burnout recovery). But, for those of you who already have burnout, I'll provide you with an evidence-based six-step recovery plan.

To do this, I'll be splitting this guide into three separate parts. In Part I we dive into understanding burnout, as we look at what burnout is (and what it isn't!), the workplace factors that cause it and the people who are most at risk. Part II is about identifying burnout, as I guide you through the Burnout Assessment Tool, so you can identify any burnout in yourself and learn ways to identify burnout in others, too. Then Part III is where we tackle recovery from burnout, and here I outline the crucial six steps to recovery, which I've grouped into three phases, as follows:

- **PHASE ONE:** Getting healthy
  - **Step 1:** Admitting there is a problem
  - **Step 2:** Distancing from work
  - **Step 3:** Restoring your health

- **PHASE TWO:** Preparing for change
  - **Step 4:** Questioning your values
  - **Step 5:** Exploring work possibilities

- **PHASE THREE:** Actioning change
  - **Step 6:** Making changes to work
  - **Bonus Step 1:** Staying healthy after change
  - **Bonus Step 2:** Identifying and overcoming barriers to change

Throughout, I've included exercises to help you engage with the material, so you can explore these as and when you feel ready and able to do so. My goal with selecting these exercises has been to ensure they are impactful but accessible and relatively quick to do.

I'll be guiding you through everything that you need to recover effectively, and stay recovered. Managing burnout is not an easy or a short process, but together we have absolutely got this!

How to use this book

Reading a book from start to finish can be overwhelming, especially when you're already feeling stressed and burned out. I've therefore broken down this guide so that it can be read sequentially, but you can also dip in and out, as needed. Feel free to start wherever feels right for you, depending on your energy levels and personal situation. However, if you'd like some guidance, then my recommendations are as follows:

- **If you work a high-stress job and you're looking for ways to keep yourself well,** I would recommend reading from the start, beginning with Part I.
- **If you're on the brink and not sure if you're burned out,** you might want to skip to Part II to work out if you are. If you're not there yet and want to work on prevention, I recommend beginning at Part I. But if you do identify as burned out, I suggest you skip straight to Part III to focus on recovery methods.

- **If you're in recovery**, you might want to go straight to Part III, where recovery is the focus. This will allow you to concentrate on the things that are most appropriate for you in the present moment.
- **If you're worried about someone else**, feel free to skip Part II, where you can learn how to identify burnout and read my advice on how you can support someone else.

My story

Before we dive in, I think it's important to share my own experience with burnout as I will be touching on this throughout the rest of the book. A warning, though: my experience of burnout has been extreme, but I want to share this with you now so that (whatever situation you're reading this from) you know that you're not alone.

I have had two burnout episodes in my life and I hope that by sharing my story you can see that if I could get through them, then so can you. I also made many mistakes along the way before I finally reached full recovery, so I'm hoping you can learn from these – and avoid the same pitfalls as me!

I first qualified as a doctor in 2008, after six years of training. I then completed ten further years of training (first in anaesthetics and then in primary care) and by 2018 I had qualified as a GP, and I took up a new position in this role. However from this point on, I very quickly developed what I now know to be burnout. At the time I had no idea what was going on because during my entire time at medical school, and during my decade of postgraduate training, the term 'burnout' had not once been mentioned. Therefore, during this time – my first burnout experience – I had absolutely no idea what was happening to me, let alone that what I was experiencing was a recognised condition with a name. All I knew, when I ended up in burnout for the first time, was that I was in a desperate state.

You might be wondering what this first burnout looked like for me. Well, during this period, I was still showing up to work and going through the motions, but internally I was a mess. My list of symptoms – both physical and mental – were extensive. I was experiencing terrible headaches and a permanent sensation of pressure on my throat, like I was choking. I was having vivid nightmares and I was exhausted, no matter how much sleep I got. I was experiencing incredibly distressing and uncontrollable intrusive thoughts, which were largely focused around harm coming to my two children. I also was incredibly negative and pessimistic and I enjoyed nothing. I had lost interest in all of my hobbies and I felt incredibly unmotivated. I was easily upset over the smallest of things, which caused problems with my family. I found I both cared too much and I felt completely numb at the same time. I had also started to self-neglect by not looking after myself physically. I struggled to make decisions at work too, as decisions that would normally have come to me easily took much longer, and I obsessed over whether I was missing things (as a doctor, this really got to me, as patient care is at the heart of what we do). My head became just the most exhausting place to exist. Yet, despite all of this, no one knew.

As I said, throughout this period I was still turning up to work and, according to feedback from colleagues at the time, I was still performing well and providing safe care for my patients. While this was a relief to hear (as I was caught up in a horrific cycle of worrying about my decision-making and decision fatigue), it meant that no one else at work had noticed that I was in crisis. I felt intense shame and loneliness as I struggled with my burnout alone, and internally I was berating myself for seemingly not being able to cope with the pressures at work.

My symptoms were significant but I forced myself to work harder in the mistaken and misguided belief that somehow I could 'work' my way out of the situation. When that didn't work I blamed myself entirely. The crunch point came when I had a panic attack, having never had one in my entire life. It shocked me into realising that I was deep into something that I couldn't control. I knew I needed to make changes at work, so I spoke to my manager and my workload was halved. I was grateful for this, but I didn't have the confidence to take what I really needed: sick leave.

I quickly realised that a reduced workload wasn't sufficient to allow me to recover, so I made the decision to leave my job. The plan was to work more flexibly while I got myself together and worked out my next career steps. At this point, I didn't know that I had burnout, but I knew there was something very wrong. I thought if I could just leave my current job then I could leave my problem behind. I referred myself to Practitioner Health (the specialist mental health service for public sector healthcare staff in the UK), but unfortunately I was not able to get an appointment before the 2020 pandemic started. I had left my job just a month before the first lockdown, and subsequently had to move fast to secure work in rapidly changing – and deeply worrying – circumstances.

During this time, I worked a variety of medical jobs and I was coping well enough now that I was distanced from the job that had burned me out. However, I was still working under very similar pressures, and I now had the additional pressure of working in healthcare during the pandemic. I could feel burnout slowly creeping back.

Looking back now, I can see I made mistakes during my first burnout, which allowed for the second burnout experience to take place. Some of these mistakes were simply because I had no idea that I was in burnout, and I just didn't know what I needed to do to recover. For instance, I didn't take any time off work (when this was an option available to me) due to the immense guilt I felt at the thought of taking sick leave, and potentially causing problems for my colleagues and patients. Other mistakes were due to circumstances that were completely out of my hands. For example, I could never have anticipated having to step up to be the sole earner for our family during the first year of the pandemic (after finally leaving the job that burned me out), but that is what was necessary at the time. After leaving the job that burned me out, I had hoped for some time to rest, recover and regroup, but instead I needed to go straight back to full-time work. I therefore didn't have the opportunity to make sufficient changes to how I worked or coped with stress, so I was vulnerable to relapse – and that's exactly what happened.

As I saw my second burnout crisis looming in 2021, I became desperate to avoid going back to that same dark place again, so I referred myself back into Practitioner Health. This time, I managed to secure myself a spot, and when I was officially diagnosed with burnout I was placed under the care of a GP and a therapist. With their support, during my second burnout experience I learned techniques and strategies to help manage my symptoms and put me on the path to recovery. The knowledge that I gained about burnout during this period helped me to identify the mistakes I had made during my first burnout experience, and I was able to correct them moving forward. For example, having not taken time off with the first, I went on to take nine months off from public sector work during my second burnout. This gave me sufficient space from the workplace factors that were fuelling my burnout, so I could engage with making the changes I needed to get better. I also went through an intense course of therapy to give me the skills to help manage the terrible anxiety I was experiencing, and to give me vital tools to help me better manage my stress.

One of the most surprising things I learned during my treatment for my second burnout was that the way I was feeling during my burnout was not down to me. Instead it was down to significant changes to the structure and function of my brain, and to changes in my stress hormones, which had a direct impact on my body. When I finally reached a point in my recovery where I had the energy to engage with reading burnout research, suddenly the pieces fell into place: I hadn't fallen apart because I wasn't good enough at coping or because there was something wrong with my stress-management skills. I had fallen apart because my brain and body had changed due to the intense stress I was under. What an absolute revelation. My symptoms were completely out of my control. That knowledge helped me to forgive myself for ending up the way I did. I hope too that by explaining this here, you might be able to find some understanding – and perhaps some forgiveness – for yourself if you are currently experiencing burnout or if you have in the past. (I will be covering the changes that happen to your brain and body in more depth in Chapter 1.)

My experience with burnout changed me, giving me a completely new perspective on life. I now work to provide burnout education to as many people as possible in a number of different ways. Online, I create digital products and social media content, and I am a medical influencer on the Fides programme for the World Health Organization (WHO), helping to combat health misinformation. As a coach and mentor, I take on individual clients to guide them through their burnout recovery and career changes, and I take on public speaking engagements to support people in this same way too. My work on burnout has been featured in publications as varied as *The Lancet* and *LADbible*.

While the career changes I've been through (as a result of my burnout) are not what I ever expected, hoped or planned for, I can safely say that the work I'm doing right now makes me happier than I've ever been. I enjoy helping to break down the stigma about burnout – and mental health generally – every day. I am forever grateful to have been given these opportunities to spread this burnout education. My mission is to continue sharing what I've learned, and my next step is to share this information with you.

AN IMPORTANT NOTE

Before we go on, I want to make clear that it's crucial to get expert help first if you identify with being in a burnout crisis or mental health crisis. This book – while written by a practising doctor – is not designed to replace medical help or guidance from a therapist. This is a guide to help you along the way with burnout prevention and recovery, and to plug the gaps that are not filled by traditional medical or psychological management of burnout.

Mental health crisis
Please consider getting urgent expert help from your doctor if you identify with any of these crisis symptoms:
- Thoughts of self-harm or suicide (please seek same-day help)
- Disabling distress or loss of function
- Significant self-neglect (for example, not washing, eating or drinking)
- Panic attacks
- Nightmares, flashbacks or hyper-vigilance
- Intrusive thoughts
- Significant sleep problems

- Careless mistakes and inability to focus
- Feeling numb, lost or out of control
- Withdrawal from relationships and socialising
- Dependence on food, alcohol or recreational drugs to cope

If you are experiencing a crisis or any of the above then, quite simply, you will not have the mental, emotional or physical capacity to read this guide and implement the changes needed on your recovery journey. Please use the precious little energy you have for getting the help you need right now, and come back for extra support from here at a later date, if needed.

Therapy

This book has been written as an adjunct to therapy, and is not designed to be a replacement for it. However, I do know that it is not easy for everyone to access therapy, so, if that's you, this guide will certainly give you some techniques and guidance to kick-start your recovery regardless. I recommend you use this book as follows:

- **If you are able to see a therapist**: The advice I share will be a fantastic add-on to the work you'll already be doing. I will take you through all the additional things you need to do outside of therapy to recover, such as looking at your career options.
- **If you are waiting to see a therapist**: This book will give you some simple therapy-based exercises and techniques to get started on while you wait. You can then continue using this advice as extra support to aid your ongoing recovery.
- **If you are unable to see a therapist**: This book will give you some simple therapy-based exercises and techniques to work with. The advice here is not intended to replace seeing a therapist, but if you have barriers to access this support, it can certainly help.

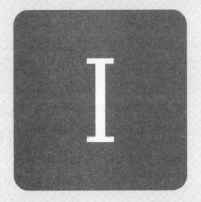

UNDERSTANDING BURNOUT

1

What is burnout?

At the height of my burnout, I was in a difficult place. My thinking slowed down and I struggled to make even simple decisions. I felt incredibly detached from the things that previously brought me joy and fulfilment, and I developed a cynicism and a level of apathy that was completely out of character for me. At my lowest point, I was so far removed from the old Claire that I didn't recognise who I was.

I did not spot the early signs of burnout and I did not realise I had a problem until it was too late – by then I'd hit crisis point. Why was this?

Quite simply, because I was never taught about burnout. During my 15 years plus of medical and postgraduate training, the concepts of burnout, stress management and how to look after yourself had never really been mentioned. As a result, when I experienced my own burnout, I didn't understand it was a recognised condition or even that it had a name.

My burnout could have been avoided if I'd had a better understanding of what it is and the signs to look out for early on, so that's what I want to share with you now. In this chapter, we'll be covering the definition of burnout and the physical and psychological symptoms to look out for. Then we'll end as I answer some of the questions that I get asked about burnout again and again. Let's begin.

Burnout: A Definition

Burnout syndrome was first described in the 1970s by a psychologist who observed that the mental distress of healthcare workers in a free HIV/AIDs clinic in New York was different to other stress-related problems that had previously been defined. However, it wasn't until 2019 (ironically the year of my own burnout) that the WHO officially recognised burnout, and gave it a definition: 'An occupational syndrome that arises as a result of prolonged workplace stress that has not been successfully managed.'

The WHO identifies three components to burnout:

1. **Depersonalisation:** The cynicism, apathy or lack of caring that develops with burnout.
2. **Emotional exhaustion:** The very real physical and emotional fatigue of caring too much for too long.
3. **Reduced professional efficacy:** Reduced performance at work.

As burnout has become a topic that more and more people are aware of, I see the term increasingly being used to describe work stress and exhaustion. You must have all three of the above components to officially have burnout syndrome, according to the WHO, although it is extremely common to identify with one or two of these components if you are at risk of or are in the early stages of sliding into burnout. If you find that you can get over work fatigue and exhaustion with a holiday or a weekend away, you most likely don't have burnout syndrome.

Most commonly, people suffering with burnout first start experiencing 'emotional exhaustion', which can present as feeling depleted, regardless of how much rest or downtime you are getting. Along with fatigue, the second most important and commonly experienced feature of burnout, according to scientists, is apathy, which would fall under 'depersonalisation'.

Burnout syndrome starts off as being reactive to your work, but eventually it will affect every single aspect of your life. So, if you feel stressed at work but you don't yet identify with all three components, this is the perfect time to act. You can make changes now to prevent things from progressing further. (If that's you, I'm so pleased you're reading this book – you're in the right place.)

Exploring the Official Burnout Definition

Before we move on, let's dig deeper into the official definition of burnout because there are a couple of things I want to draw your attention to.

First, it's interesting to note that the WHO definition does not state that burnout is a mental or medical health problem; instead they classify burnout as an 'occupational syndrome'. Whether or not burnout should be recognised as a medical or mental health problem is highly debated within the scientific community. But, as far as the WHO is concerned, they do not consider burnout to be a mental health problem because it is entirely reactive to environmental pressures.

My personal take on this is that there are plenty of medical problems that are reactive to the environment; for example, the vast majority of lung cancer cases are caused by environmental exposure to cigarette smoke. We also know that asthma patients have more poorly controlled symptoms when they are exposed to high levels of air pollution, as another example. As we learn more, you will come to understand – as I did – that burnout causes pathological changes to the brain and body with a defined set of signs and symptoms and a recognised recovery process. To my mind, as a doctor with many years of clinical experience, this all sounds very much like burnout is a medical or mental health problem. However, I also fully admit that I carry a fair amount of bias when it comes to the definition, having experienced burnout myself. Therefore, you will notice during this book that I will often talk about burnout as if it is a medical or mental health problem, but please know that this is not the official definition.

Second, you will notice that the official definition focuses on burnout as occurring in the workplace only. However, this approach fails to recognise the stress caused by unpaid labour, such as that done by carers or parents. It also fails to recognise that burnout can also occur outside of the workplace for certain groups of people, such as those with attention-deficit hyperactivity disorder (ADHD) or autism (more on this on p. 80). Therefore, I personally disagree with this aspect of the definition as I certainly believe that burnout can occur beyond the workplace.

In workplace burnout, the cause of the burnout is the workplace stress you're under. But one of the difficulties with carer or parental burnout is that you have very little control over the source and nature of your stress, so it is difficult to remove yourself from it.

With parenting, of course, your children will grow and develop, and the stressors that you are under will change over time. I no longer have to worry, for example, about keeping my toddlers from killing themselves by sprinting towards a busy road with no warning, but now they're older we have the stresses of friendships, hormones and emotional changes instead.

With caring, whether or not things change over time for the better or for the worse entirely depends on each individual situation. For example, this will depend on whether you are caring for elderly relatives or perhaps for people with progressive illnesses; the prognosis; the level of dependency required by the person you are caring for; and many other factors.

Parents and carers usually work long hours and are not well supported by the systems in society today, financially or otherwise. This is all complicated by the intense emotions involved in parenting and caring and, for the most part, there will be huge amounts of love involved too. However, love alone will not prevent burnout in the context of huge and sustained stress, and parenting and caring provide the perfect storm for burnout to occur.

Carers and parents, if you are reading this, please know that I see you and I recognise that burnout is a problem that you face. The advice and suggestions that I give in this book will be focused on work but they are still applicable to you. On top of this, my advice to you is to work on improving how you perceive your caring duties, and I encourage you to engage in therapy and make small changes to how you are physically supported, where you can.

Now we know what burnout is, let's look at how it shows up in real terms in the form of physical and psychological symptoms.

If you are feeling massively burned out right now, then learning about how profoundly the brain and body change as a result of your burnout might not be helpful for you in this moment. If this is you, please skip to Chapter 2 for now and re-read this section when you are feeling better in yourself. I personally found it a relief to know that my symptoms were as a result of these changes, but I totally understand that others might not have the same experience. Be kind to yourself if you're unsure and come back to this at another time when you have a little more capacity.

Physical Symptoms of Burnout

Let's start with the physical symptoms of burnout. These can show up as:

- Chest pain
- Palpitations
- Stomach pain
- Bloating
- Shortness of breath
- Headaches
- Dizziness
- Increased minor illnesses and reduced immunity
- Poor sleep
- Appetite changes (increased or decreased)
- Muscle tension and pain
- High blood pressure
- Fatigue
- Irregular periods
- Very low or high libido

This is not an exhaustive list. One of my burned-out colleagues ground their teeth so much from stress that they actually broke a tooth! I've also had people tell me they experience significant neurological symptoms, such as numbness and pins and needles. My own physical symptoms were predominately: headaches, shoulder and neck pain, a choking-like sensation on the front of my neck, nightmares, poor-quality sleep, and fatigue that was completely disproportionate to the amount of sleep I was (or wasn't) getting. Everyone experiences their physical burnout symptoms differently.

Why are Physical Symptoms so Common in Burnout?

When we get stressed and our brain detects a threat, our bodies produce stress hormones including adrenaline and cortisol. This stress hormone response is designed to deal with immediate and short-term threats, and it allows the body to go into 'fight or flight' mode. When 'flight or fight' is activated, we experience all the physical changes we associate with this, such as the heart rate going up and the breath quickening. During this time, our body prioritises 'fight or flight' over anything else, such as maintaining the immune, reproductive or digestive systems.

In the early days of humanity, our stress response and 'fight or flight' mode was important to help protect us from physical threats, such as a lion appearing on the horizon. We have evolved over time, and in the modern world our stress response tends to be activated more frequently by perceived or emotional threats (such as doing a presentation or opening an email) rather than physical threats. For some people who are burned out, or slipping into burnout, simply walking into your place of work might become considered a perceived threat, enough to trigger your body's stress response. This would mean that by simply walking into your office, your 'fight or flight' mode could be activated, causing your heart to start pounding and a feeling of overwhelm. Regardless of what the threat is, the body's stress response is still the same because it does not know the difference between a physical and a perceived threat.

If your stress is short-lived and not too intense, a little bit of adrenaline and cortisol can, in fact, be helpful – even in the modern world. Think about the last time you sat an exam. This is a great example of a situation where you were likely to have felt under some short-lived stress, and the extra adrenaline and cortisol could have produced beneficial effects for you, such as improved concentration, focus and performance. Your stress response being activated in this situation allows you to perform well under pressure.

However, if your stress response is prolonged or too intense it can become harmful – this is what we see in burnout, as your 'fight or flight' mode can become consistently activated. At this point, your stress hormones stop being the helpful, short-term response to a threat that they are designed for. Instead, this chronic activation of 'fight or flight' makes the body's response to stress change from being potentially helpful to unhelpful and harmful. We are, quite simply, not designed to live in a state of chronic and intense stress.

As we've discussed, when you live in a permanent state of 'fight or flight' your body prioritises this response over and above anything else, and this can trigger physical symptoms of burnout. For example, as your body neglects your digestive system, gut problems can occur; as your body neglects your immune system, you might find yourself getting ill more frequently; or as your body makes your heart beat faster for long periods of time, you might develop palpitations or shortness of breath. This is why physical symptoms are so common in burnout.

I would strongly advise those of you that are experiencing any physical symptoms to seek medical advice, and to be assessed for alternative causes for your symptoms other than burnout. For instance, as mentioned above, palpitations are a common symptom of burnout due to activation of your 'fight or flight' response. However, palpitations can also be caused by other problems, and so your doctor will likely want to do some tests to find out the cause. Similarly, fatigue is a core symptom of burnout, but if you're feeling tired all the time then it's definitely worthwhile ruling out any alternative cause of your symptoms, such as anaemia or thyroid problems. It's common to have normal medical test results in burnout, but please go through the process of eliminating alternative causes for your symptoms first!

Burnout and the Risk of Significant Health Complications

For some people with burnout, the body moves on from the 'flight or fight' mode and they begin to experience something called an 'adaptive' or 'altered' stress response instead. This is important to know because this adaptive stress response can cause problems for long-term health. Let me explain.

For people with an adaptive stress response, you'll initially see a rise in stress hormones but then, with time, the body adapts and you see a *fall* in stress hormones. When your stress hormone levels start to fall, your risk of problems such as high blood pressure and heart disease increases. This can be difficult to get your head around because you might think that a drop in stress hormones would be good for the body after a period of them being high. However, when your stress hormones drop this significantly, in the context of ongoing stress, it triggers low-grade inflammation in the body, and it's this inflammation that is thought to be one of the reasons for these long-term problems (such as the high blood pressure and heart disease, as mentioned).

Sticking with heart problems, one study followed burnout patients for nearly 25 years. Within this group there was a 20 per cent increased risk of atrial fibrillation (i.e. a problem with the rhythm of the heart) that can cause strokes if left untreated. Also, employees scoring in the top 20 per cent on the burnout scale at baseline had a whopping 79 per cent increased risk of being diagnosed with coronary heart disease over a three-year period. The authors of this study speculated that the stresses of a grinding workday may be 'just as detrimental as lighting up a cigarette or eating a double bacon cheeseburger!' This is a hugely significant statement to make about the physical risks of burnout.

The underlying mechanisms about how burnout increases your chance of heart problems are not completely understood, though. Researchers think that the altered stress response is one of the causes, as already mentioned above, but that's not the full story. Heart problems in burnout are also thought to be linked to metabolic syndrome, sleep disorders, reduced immunity and changes to how your blood clots with chronic stress.

It's speculated that the adoption of poor health behaviours, such as smoking and a lack of physical activity, by those that burn out also factors into the increased risk. Poor food habits can also be a factor, as 56 per cent of burned-out doctors reported changing food habits – either eating less because they were too busy or forgetful, or eating more for comfort. Certainly, when I was hugely burned out, I wasn't eating properly because I simply wasn't motivated and I didn't have the energy to do so. I also wasn't exercising or sleeping properly. On occasion, I didn't even have the energy to brush my teeth or wash my face. In fact, during my burnout, my self-neglect was quite significant. It's easy enough to believe that form of self-neglect and poor health behaviours over a prolonged period of time can become risk factors for cardiovascular problems.

It's not just your heart that suffers when you're burned out; you're more likely to be involved in a serious accident too. In fact, if you are under the age of 45 and you burn out, you have an increased risk of dying prematurely from any cause. Burnout can cause a huge range of physical symptoms and additional health risks because of the changes it makes to your brain and normal physiology. The following physical consequences have been found by scientists to be significantly linked with burnout:

- Type 2 diabetes
- High cholesterol
- Coronary artery disease
- Hospitalisation for cardiovascular disease
- Musculoskeletal pain (overall pain, neck-shoulder pain, back pain and pain-related disability)
- Fatigue
- Headaches
- Respiratory infections
- Stomach problems

- Severe injuries
- Increased risk of death from all causes if under the age of 45

You are also more likely to have depressive symptoms and are at higher risk of being admitted for a mental health problem. If this comes as news to you, then please be reassured that I certainly had no realisation as to how risky burnout is for physical health when I was going through it. Looking back, I find it so incredibly hard to think that, as a doctor, I had not realised the seriousness of it, even though my physical symptoms were significant.

Former tech co-founder and Head of Engineering, Dan Bartlett (37) (https://danbartlett.co.uk and https://nobt.co.uk) describes his physical symptoms of early burnout:

Physical exhaustion. The fatigue was quite intense at times. I'd feel exhausted by 11am and then push through the rest of the day with caffeine, alcohol and adrenaline. Some mornings, I'd feel like I could sleep for 12 hours. Yet at the end of the day, it would take me hours to fall asleep. My eyes in particular felt almost bruised, and there was a deep ache throughout my chest.

Everyone experiences burnout slightly differently. It's helpful to know what your own physical symptoms are so that you can track their improvement through your recovery process and use them as a means of monitoring if you are slipping backwards again (i.e. if your symptoms worsen). The following exercise will help you to do this.

Exercise 1

Identify your physical symptoms

If you are currently experiencing burnout, or feeling like you are slipping down that path, write down all of your physical symptoms now. Keep this list somewhere safe but accessible, for easy reference in the future so you can monitor your symptoms.

Psychological Symptoms of Burnout

How would you feel if I were to tell you that the reason why you cannot handle your emotions like you used to, or you get overwhelmed with seemingly small, insignificant triggers, or you've slowed down and struggle with concentration is all because of structural and functional changes to your brain caused by burnout?

While I totally get that for some people hearing that burnout can cause these changes might sound scary, the good news is that we don't think these changes are permanent, so don't panic! For me, knowing about the psychological symptoms of burnout and how they are founded in genuine brain changes (i.e. they occurred outside of my conscious control) has liberated me from so much guilt, so I hope this might help you too. You see, psychological changes start slowly and build, but here's the kicker – often you're not consciously aware of it until you hit a burnout crisis.

During my burnout, I would often sit at work in my surgery and internally berate myself for struggling with tasks that I would previously have sailed through. I beat myself up for struggling with extreme decision fatigue, or I'd end up in tears because of an unexpected email or request that I felt unable to handle. Looking back now, I know it would have been so helpful to understand that the reason I couldn't cope with these tasks was not because of my abilities but because my brain had changed. In other words, how I was feeling wasn't my fault. All the intrusive thoughts, all the worry, all the ruminating, all the emotional dysregulation... none of it was anything I could have controlled consciously. No amount of self-blame, yoga or bubble baths was going to be enough to help me feel better in my head or change how slow and laboured my thinking had become during my burnout. Neither my degree in neuroscience nor my subsequent years in medical training and practice had ever touched on this vital information, so that's why I want to share it with you now.

Let's start by talking about some of the psychological symptoms of burnout. These include:

- Difficulty sleeping (can also be a physical symptom)
- Low mood
- Anxiety
- Worry
- Cynicism
- Detachment
- Irritability
- Anger outbursts
- Forgetfulness or poor memory
- Poor concentration
- Decision fatigue
- Difficulty problem solving

Dan Bartlett describes the psychological symptoms of burnout he experienced:

A lot of the time I felt numb, yet frequently close to tears; juggling many complex ideas, yet unable to focus on one thing; knowing I needed a break but unable to escape. The most simple tasks became gargantuan struggles. I felt incompetent and unproductive, like I was letting others down.

The scariest symptoms for me were a kind of detachment and derealisation. It would feel like I couldn't take anything more in, and I'd start to dissociate from what was happening. This was alarming and made me very anxious. I also felt so alone. Outside, everyone was cheering me on. The company was doing well. But internally I felt disconnected and distant. Why was I struggling so much?

My own psychological symptoms manifested themselves in struggling to maintain attention and stay focused while problem solving. I found it hard to make fast, simple decisions about the management of my patients, whereas pre-burnout my decision-making was quicker and immediately off the top of my head. I still came to the same decisions, but it required a lot more effort and time to get there. The slowing down of thinking and 'brain fog' are how some people describe this, and it contributed to my reduced performance at work (or 'reduced professional efficacy' if we were to refer back to the three components of burnout as described by the WHO, *see* p. 19).

The Science Behind Psychological Symptoms

If you're interested in the detailed science behind these psychological symptoms, then here's the geeky bit. Burnout causes the amygdala (the part of your brain that is involved in emotional regulation and fear responses) to get bigger. During burnout, you also experience weakened connections between the amygdala and other areas of the brain involved in emotional regulations. In particular, you get a weakened connection between the amygdala and the medial prefrontal cortex, which is where you process a lot of higher-level thinking and functioning that can help control some of the input from the amygdala. But these weakened connections in burnout mean the brain is less able to suppress the amygdala and its fear responses, so you experience increased levels of fear as you experience burnout.

As well as weakened connections, burnout causes thinning and early ageing of the medial prefrontal cortex. This means that this part of the brain ages more rapidly than if you didn't have burnout, worsening any psychological symptoms you might be experiencing. In addition, you see significant reductions in volumes of grey matter (the part of your brain and nervous system that is composed of your nerve cell bodies and their branches) in the areas of the brain responsible for memory, attention and emotional difficulties. Grey matter plays a crucial role in allowing you to function day to day, so when you start to lose it in these areas, your symptoms or poor memory, poor attention and emotional dysregulation get worse.

Take it from someone that is a bit of a neuroscience geek: the changes that happen in your brain during burnout are real and they are significant. In fact, these changes due to burnout are really similar to the changes that we see as a result of other problems such as post-traumatic stress disorder (PTSD) and survivors of adverse childhood events, so they're not to be downplayed. Ultimately, too, the worse your burnout, the bigger the changes in your brain.

Some Good News

The happier news is that the changes to your brain that occur during burnout can be reversed. In lab studies, the brains of stressed rats return to normal structure and function when stress is removed. Similarly, with medical students studying for exams, the stress that is seen to cause structural and functional changes in the brain during this period is reversed by four weeks after the exam is done.

Cognitive behavioural therapy (CBT) (*see* p. 133) for burnout has been found to reduce the size of the amygdala and return the prefrontal cortex to normal. We also have evidence that acceptance and commitment therapy (ACT) (*see* p. 136) is useful in the treatment of burnout. In other words, therapy can change your brain's function and structure. There is much more to full burnout recovery, of course (as we'll address in Part III), but what an incredible thing to know that these psychological symptoms can be reversed and that talking therapies can help.

What I hope you are getting from this section is an understanding of why you feel the way that you do, if you're feeling burnt out. I hope that with this understanding comes a sense of empowerment through knowing that you're not stuck, even if you feel like you are, as your symptoms *can* be reversed. How you're feeling now doesn't have to be a permanent state. I want to make it clear that it's not your fault that you're feeling the way that you do. So many people with burnout end up with very severe symptoms, having not recognised the slide into burnout until it is too late. I'm one of those people, so believe me when I say there is absolutely no judgement here if this happened to you too.

Perhaps, like me, you realised that there was something wrong but you were either in denial (the denial is strong!) or you threw yourself into working harder in a misguided attempt to fix things. Whatever your situation, the important point now is to begin taking note of any psychological symptoms you experience from this moment on, so here's two exercises to help you to start doing just that.

Exercise 2

Identify your psychological symptoms

Write down your psychological symptoms to keep alongside the list of your physical symptoms you noted on p. 27. These can be used to monitor improvements and to catch yourself if you are slipping back into burnout.

Exercise 3

Identify how your behaviour has changed

Imagine that a camera crew have followed you around, filming your every move. How did you end up acting differently because of burnout? What differences would be picked up on camera? Think about changes both at work and at home.

If you're stuck, think about how you interact with others and your working habits and patterns. Also think about your coping mechanisms (both healthy and unhealthy), such as movement, smoking, eating, drinking or use of other substances. Keep this list safe, too, so you can monitor any changes.

BURNOUT WITH ANXIETY AND DEPRESSION

Around 60 per cent of people with burnout have a concurrent mental health problem, like anxiety or depression. I want to include a special mention of burnout in relation to anxiety and depression here because of how often they are linked.

It can be confusing for the burned-out person (and sometimes for the healthcare professionals helping them with their recovery) to make the distinction between burnout and anxiety or depression, particularly as the definitions and the experience of anxiety and depression can feel very similar to burnout and often the treatments given are also the same.

However, when it comes to burnout recovery, it doesn't simply mean having therapy and potentially taking antidepressants. The recovery for burnout is much more involved and complex than taking a purely medical or psychological approach (as we'll see in Part III). So, making the distinction between burnout and anxiety and depression here is helpful for guiding you through your burnout management. We'll look at each in turn.

Anxiety

Everyone worries. Intermittent worry and periodic anxiety is a totally normal thing to experience. It's when it starts to persistently affect function, performance at work and/or relationships that it becomes a mental health problem, rather than part of the normal human experience. Symptoms of generalised anxiety, which can cause significant distress and affect the sufferer's function, both at home and at work, might include:

- Long-term excessive worry that is unrelated to particular circumstances
- Sleep problems
- Heart palpitations
- Poor concentration
- Restlessness
- Irritability

Many of the symptoms of anxiety overlap with those of burnout; however, the distinction is generally found in the history of symptom development, as often people with generalised anxiety are not able to pinpoint a cause. Also, in burnout, you have the additional feature of depersonalisation (i.e. feeling cynical and apathetic), which is not typically a feature in anxiety.

Depression

When screening for depression, a doctor might ask the following questions:

- During the last month, have you often been bothered by feeling down, depressed or hopeless?
- During the last month, have you often been bothered by having little interest or pleasure in doing things?

If the patient answers 'yes' to one of the questions and the symptoms have been present most days, most of the time, for at least two weeks, then the doctor might move on to ask about associated symptoms of depression, such as:

- Disturbed sleep (decreased or increased compared to usual)
- Decreased or increased appetite and/or weight
- Fatigue or loss of energy
- Agitation or slowing down of movements and thoughts
- Poor concentration or indecisiveness
- Feelings of worthlessness or excessive or inappropriate guilt
- Recurrent thoughts of death, recurrent suicidal ideas, or a suicide attempt or specific plan

As with anxiety, you can see that often the symptoms of depression are very similar to burnout. However, in depression, typically the symptoms do not start as related to work alone, and most people with depression do not go through the five stages of burnout (as outlined on p. 96). You will also notice that depersonalisation (one of the three core features of burnout, see p. 19) does not feature in the definition of depression. However, to complicate matters slightly, for those that end up in burnout and progress to habitual burnout – the fifth stage of burnout – depression is commonly seen and diagnosed (see p. 100 for more detail on this).

It can therefore be confusing to work out if you have depression, depression and burnout, or solely burnout. It is entirely possible that you might start with burnout alone, but then progress to depression if your burnout is not successfully managed. I recommend that you speak to your doctor for clarification if you are unsure.

Common Questions about Burnout

Before we move on, I thought it'd be useful if I address some of the same questions about burnout that I get asked again and again.

Are antidepressants helpful in burnout?
Some surveys suggest around 40 per cent of workers with burnout are prescribed antidepressant medication, and having burnout means you are more likely to be prescribed antidepressants, too. Going on to antidepressants is an individual decision – one that needs to be discussed with your doctor. Normally, your doctor would consider giving you antidepressants for moderate to severe anxiety or depression (which often run alongside burnout), but *burnout alone is not an indication for antidepressants*. If you don't have depression or anxiety alongside burnout, antidepressants are not going to be helpful in the long run.

If you're confused about whether you have anxiety, depression, burnout or a combination, speak to a doctor for their assessment and advice.

If you're already on antidepressants, please do not stop them suddenly, as doing this could make you very unwell. Please speak to your doctor before making any medication changes.

Can you tell me more about the lack of teaching on burnout in formal medical education and its impact?
Despite an increased awareness of the phenomenon of burnout, there is still a lack of understanding about it among the medical profession. This is partly due to the WHO only having recognised burnout as a syndrome since 2019, and a general lack of training on burnout in medical curriculums.

At no point during my medical training was burnout discussed, mentioned or taught. Literally nothing. Nothing during medical school and nothing during my postgraduate training. For context, I started my medical training in 2002 and I became a GP at the end of 2018. For myself, I don't recall ever being given a diagnosis of burnout when I was at the height of it all... it's just something that I eventually worked out for myself.

How can you be given a diagnosis when your doctor might be completely unaware of the problem or hasn't been taught about it? It's not possible.

Given the huge burden of burnout right now (it really is the post-pandemic pandemic), my personal belief is that doctors need to upskill themselves on what burnout is and (crucially) how to appropriately support patients with it. The good news is that I genuinely do think this is happening. I am encouraged to see that a lot of my peers are now much more aware of what burnout is and how to support their burned-out patients. Burnout recovery is hard and long, and a purely medical approach is not enough. Doctors need to know this so that they can signpost their patients to the right support.

Why can burnout be difficult to diagnose?
We have the perfect storm of doctors not being aware of or taught about burnout in addition to the fact that burnout itself is difficult to diagnose. Many symptoms of burnout overlap with those of anxiety, depression, PTSD and some physical health problems too.

The other complicating factor is that quite often burnout comes hand in hand with other diagnoses, so making the distinction between different problems or symptoms can be confusing for both doctors and patients. However, there are tools that can be used to help diagnose burnout, which I will share later in the book (*see* p. 96*).*

Is burnout even a medical problem?
Burnout is officially recognised and defined as an occupational syndrome rather than as a medical or mental health problem. This might go some way to explaining why you might have difficulties getting diagnosed with 'burnout'. If it isn't recognised as a medical problem then why would you or your doctor even think to consider it as a diagnosis?

The semantics of the definition are debatable. Burnout definitely causes pathological changes to the brain and body. We know from studies that there are changes to the size, structure and function of the brain (a 'signature hallmark', no less) due to burnout, as well as changes to the neuroendocrine system. We also know that these changes are reversible with time and treatment. To my mind, that begs the question: Is it right to categorise burnout as an occupational syndrome rather than a mental health problem?

This is where it gets a bit murky. The changes to the brain and the body with burnout are different to those of other mental health problems, such as depression and anxiety. In fact, you see depression and anxiety in nearly 60 per cent of people with burnout, meaning that about 40 per cent of people with burnout *do not* have those mental health problems alongside their burnout. Rather confusingly, though, a lot of the symptoms overlap, which makes it tricky for both doctors and patients to distinguish between them.

One concern about recategorising burnout as anything other than an occupational syndrome is that it makes burnout a problem for the individual to solely solve and relieves the burden of change and responsibility for the employer.

Essentially, my view is that – regardless of its classification – I think you can absolutely argue that burnout can be diagnosed. Doctors should give the diagnosis as appropriate, and signpost people to appropriate help too.

Chapter 1 Takeaways

- A little stress, in short bursts, can be helpful for your performance and productivity, but chronic stress can lead to burnout.
- Burnout causes significant, wide-ranging physical symptoms due to the activation of stress hormones.
- Burnout also causes increased risks of a large variety of health problems and conditions, including heart problems and increased risk of dying of any cause under the age of 45.
- The reasons for increased health risks and problems are not completely understood. They are largely due to the way the body changes and adapts to burnout, as well as how our health behaviours change with burnout.

- The problems you have with reduced attention, difficulty focusing, decision fatigue, poor memory and controlling your emotional response to stress are all because your burned-out brain has changed structure and function.
- The bigger the amount of stress that you are under at work, the bigger the changes in your brain and body and the worse you will feel as a result.
- You may have features of other primary mental health problems, such as anxiety or depression, but this is not always the case.
- The good news is that the problems you are experiencing and the changes to your body and brain are reversible, but this takes time and hard work.

Workplace factors that cause burnout

As per the official WHO definition (*see* p. 19), burnout is a workplace problem caused by long-term and sustained stress that has not been successfully managed. So, the environment we work in has a huge impact on whether we suffer from burnout or not. There are six specific workplace factors that have been identified as causing burnout, and we'll explore each one in turn in this chapter. These six factors are:

1. Control
2. Reward
3. Values
4. Community
5. Fairness
6. Workload

It's been found that burnout can be caused by a problem with just one or more of these factors in your working environment. That's right, just one. That's all it takes.

Now, I appreciate that very few of us are fortunate enough to have control over our company culture and working environment, so you might be wondering why we're discussing this now. It's important to understand these six factors because they form a key aspect of both effective burnout prevention and recovery.

If you are currently working in a high-stress job, for example, but you don't think you're at burnout yet, knowing the workplace factors that put you at higher risk means that you can target any changes you make directly towards avoiding issues with these to better protect yourself. Similarly, if you think that you are currently burned out, it is essential that you identify the factors in the workplace that caused your burnout in the first place. Otherwise, if you try to continue as normal without making sufficient changes, these factors will still be there and they will cause you to burn out again. Without a doubt, knowledge is power when it comes to burnout. If you are able to successfully identify what is and isn't working for you (after reading this chapter), this is key information to be used when taking stock of your job or considering a change.

If you are lucky enough to be in charge of your company culture (for instance, if you are in a leadership role or in HR), you could use the information in this chapter to help you make impactful changes to your workplace. The structural and systemic causes of burnout must be addressed by management to help with both burnout prevention and recovery more broadly. If you change workplace burnout culture, you will stop employees from burning out in the first place. Like most physical health problems, such as strokes or heart attacks, prevention is so much easier and more cost efficient than cure.

EVERY EXPERIENCE IS INDIVIDUAL

Although burnout appears as a result of workplace culture, not everyone who experiences the working culture I'm about to describe will be affected by burnout. This is because you can put a group of people in the same working environment with the same (or similar) roles, and some will burn out while others will not. Some individuals, due to prior experiences and personality types, will be more or less at risk of burning out than others (we explore this further in Chapter 3).

As you explore the six workplace factors that cause burnout, work through the exercises for each. These are specifically written to empower you to make changes at work and to get you thinking about how to prevent burnout (if you realise you're at risk) or how to manage your recovery effectively if you're already there. (We'll have a more in-depth look at burnout recovery tools in Part III, *see* p. 109.)

1. Control

A sense of control (or perceived control) at work is essential for both burnout prevention and recovery.

To give an example, I recently delivered a webinar on burnout to a group of HR professionals. This group of hard-working professionals are currently at high risk of burnout due to a number of factors that leave them feeling very 'out of control' at work. These include: an increasingly large and complex stack of caseloads that keeps growing; a lack of appropriate training; and a lack of adequate support from management (who themselves are also struggling with the same difficulties). This situation is further compounded as some colleagues are forced to take sick leave due to stress (having worked until they cannot physically continue any longer), leaving their caseloads to be picked up by the remaining colleagues.

In a situation like this, I think it's easy to see how a lack of control at work could lead to overwhelm and burnout, if it were to continue for a long period of time. It's also easy to see how the individuals in this case study would feel powerless when it comes to their ability to create change in their working culture to ease any of these pressures.

You will always have control over *some* aspects of your work – it is important to remind yourself of this. To use this same HR example, the individuals might find control in this situation by asking for more training and supervision, by actively seeking out peer support and safe spaces to offload, or by being more proactive in organising their diaries to ensure their breaks are always protected. What works for them might not be control over the larger pressures, but they may be able to take control over some of the smaller issues instead.

The crucial point here is that control over the small things is just as effective as control over the bigger things when it comes to burnout. Ultimately, control is control! So, even if you can't control the things that you might *want* to, remembering that you do have some agency over your situation can help at times when you might otherwise feel powerless. If exercising control or autonomy is something that you are finding hard in your work right now, the following exercise is a really useful way to help you identify which aspects of your work you *are* able to control.

Exercise 4

The circle of control

Grab a pen and an A4 piece of paper and draw two concentric circles on it.

In the largest/outer circle, write down your list of concerns about your current work (or life). This is your *circle of concerns*.

When you've filled in the larger circle, go through each item again and write down in the smaller/inner circle those things from the larger circle that you have some influence or direct control over. This is your *circle of control*.

Write down all of your work stresses and concerns, and put them into the appropriate circles.

To give an example, one of your concerns might be your current workload, and you're thinking of ways to try to manage this. Some solutions will be within your circle of control; others will not. For instance, in the inner circle (the circle of control) you might write: 'email my manager to arrange a meeting to discuss my workload'. In the outer circle (the circle of concerns), you might write, 'my manager's response to my email'.

The aim of this exercise is to let go and release the things that you cannot control (i.e. those written in the largest circle). Trying to fight these concerns will mean you expend a lot of energy on something where you are not likely to be successful. Focus instead on the concerns in the smallest circle. Which factor in the smallest circle do you want to work on first?

The reason why control matters – even if it is only perceived control – is because anyone who believes that they have this control then goes on to proactively change their behaviours and their work environments to help themselves and their burnout.

However, it's also important to remember that the small elements of control might not, in themselves, be enough to entirely protect the individual from burnout. Employers really should be taking responsibility for this if the problem is within their organisation, particularly if they want to genuinely create an anti-burnout culture.

I also want to acknowledge that there are sections of society who, for structural reasons, find gaining control very hard because they are both traditionally and systemically denied it. I'm talking about people who are discriminated against or encounter bias because of factors like their race, ethnicity or sexuality. In these cases, the small wins and perceived control really matters. If this is you, then the lack of control being denied to you is grossly unfair. But, remember, even if the only things you have direct control over are as small or as simple as how you communicate your boundaries or when you take your lunch break, this exercise is still a great reminder that you can always find something that you have control over.

2. Reward

Another workplace factor that can lead to burnout is a decreased sense of reward. You might well think of your work 'reward' as your financial compensation, but your sense of reward isn't purely about how much you get paid. Rather, it includes things such as getting positive feedback, being supported to develop professionally and being given new opportunities in the workplace, as well as your own internal sense of reward by being able to engage in personally meaningful work. Cumulatively, these things all factor together to build a culture of reward.

When you feel that you are rewarded fairly for your work, or when you find your daily work rewarding in itself, your chances of burning out are significantly reduced. Conversely, if you often feel that you are not adequately rewarded for the work you do, you may be at more risk of burnout.

While pay isn't the sole mechanism of feeling rewarded at work, it does remain an important part. This is particularly true for those groups that still experience barriers in society that systemically prevent access to fair and equitable pay. For instance, the gender pay gap means that women effectively work two months of every year for free as compared to their male counterparts. In England, women hospital doctors still earn on average 18.9 per cent less than men based on a comparison of full-time equivalent mean pay, and this gap exists even after being adjusted for age, seniority and other factors. What this means is that across her lifetime, on average, a woman will earn £260,000 less than a man in the same occupation in the UK – but for higher earning professions this figure can go into the millions. The gender pay gap means that reduced financial reward is one of the multiple reasons that women in the workplace are at higher risk of burnout than men (more on this on p. 89).

Types of Rewards

Rewards within the workplace can be viewed as formal or informal and extrinsic or intrinsic:

* **Formal rewards** would be things like official awards, your employer funding a course to help with professional development, and your pay cheque.
* **Informal rewards** are things like a quick email to give you some good feedback or a meeting where someone acknowledges one of your wins.

- **Extrinsic (external) rewards** are ones that are given to you by others, such as your manager.
- **Intrinsic (internal) rewards** are all about how meaningful the work is for you, i.e. your own internal reward for the work that you do. For example, a teacher might find it rewarding to see a struggling student start to make progress as a result of their input.

This intrinsic (or internal) reward is important because meaningful work has a deep impact on burnout prevention. It's been found that you need to spend just 20 per cent of your time at work doing personally meaningful work in order to reduce your burnout risk by half. Spending 20 per cent of your time on this is the sweet spot, which I believe is very achievable. For context, if you work five days a week, that would equate to one day of personally meaningful work. In an eight-hour work day, that would equate to one hour and forty minutes being spent on personally meaningful work.

Personally meaningful work is just that: work that means something to you personally. For some people that might mean customer interactions; for others it might be teaching or product development. To identify your own personally meaningful work, think about when you've had a really good day at work and when you've felt really uplifted by it. What were you doing? What was it about that work that gave you fire in your belly?

Exercise 5

Rewards at work – journal prompts
Use the journal prompts below to help you understand and identify the rewards that work for you:
- What makes you feel the most rewarded at work? (For example, if you work in retail, you might write down how good it makes you feel when you provide excellent customer service to a disgruntled customer.)

- Are there things that could be done differently to make you feel more rewarded? (For example, would you like more feedback from your manager or extra training to feel like your company is investing in you?)
- How could you ask for change? (For example, is there a manager or team member that you could approach with your concerns? Would it be best to go with other members of your team? Would it be better to communicate via email or in person?)
- What does personally meaningful work mean to you? (Think about a time you felt uplifted at work and what triggered this.)
- Are there any ways that you could tweak your job description or do some professional development in order to hit that sweet spot of spending 20 per cent of your time at work doing things that are personally meaningful?

3. Values

When it comes to values, there are two factors that directly influence the development of burnout: the alignment of your personal values with those of your organisation and the feeling of being valued by your employer.

The Alignment of Your Personal Values with those of Your Organisation

If there is a mismatch between the two, you run the risk of burnout.

For example, you may value your work-life balance and enjoy pursuing interests outside of work, but your employer might have a corporate work culture that values long hours and expects employees to be routinely and immediately available outside of normal working hours. In this instance there is a mismatch of values that will cause stress and can lead to burnout.

Another example would be if you personally value sustainability and social responsibility, but your employer prioritises profit over these values. In this instance, you will be at risk of burnout due to the stress of the internal conflict that will arise from this mismatch.

Finally, you might value innovation and creativity but work in an organisation that values structure and process. In this instance, burnout can arise due to stress caused by low fulfilment, frustration and the lack of creative work.

The Feeling of Being Valued by Your Employer

This is a protective factor against burnout. Often it's the small things that make a big difference to how you feel about your work: that quick email to give you some positive feedback; your boss taking the time to let you know about a development opportunity that would be perfect for you; or being offered flexible working, for example. Being valued and listened to is important in the workplace. If you don't get the sense of being valued by your employer, then you will be at risk of burnout even if you love your job and your work is intrinsically meaningful or rewarding to you.

HOW CAN YOU BURN OUT FROM A JOB YOU LOVE?

One of the things people often find interesting is that you can love your job – and it can bring you immense personal value – but you can still burn out. Hence why we still see so many people in vocational jobs (which can carry a lot of personal meaning and value) burn out.

This is explained by something called the Motivation-Hygiene Theory, which states that the things that motivate us at work (i.e. the things that bring us value) exist completely independently of the things that don't (these things that don't motivate us are the so-called 'hygiene factors').

The elements that might motivate people and bring value to their work may include the work itself, opportunities for advancement, recognition, performance and achievement, job status, responsibility and personal growth.

The hygiene factors that often dissatisfy people may include:

- Salary
- Working conditions
- The physical workspace
- Relationships with colleagues and seniors
- Policies and rules

These hygiene factors are described as being like pebbles that grind us down over time. This is because these things can be tolerated in small doses only. Over time, they can build up to outweigh the personal satisfaction and value, and this can lead to burnout.

In medicine, for example, without a doubt the job itself is incredibly satisfying and rewarding. Even though I have experienced burnout as a doctor, I have never finished a day of work and thought that I hadn't made a positive impact on someone's life as a result of my input, which I value greatly. But this alone was not enough to protect me from burnout. Prolonged stress at work combined with problems with the working conditions (i.e. my workplace hygiene factors) became so overwhelming that loving the work itself – and gaining great personal value from it – was just not sufficient enough to protect me from burnout.

Exercise 6

Being valued at work – journal prompts
Use these journal prompts to reflect on your values alignment with your employer:

- What are your personal values? (If you're unsure, skip ahead to p. 144 to work these out first.)
- What are your employer's values?
- Are there any conflicts between what you value personally and how you are expected to work? If so, how does this make you feel about your work?

The following will help you reflect on feeling valued by your employer:

- In an ideal world, what would your employer do to make you feel valued at work?
- What work do you find the most valuable?
- How often are you able to do this type of work?
- What hygiene factors directly impact on your experience of being valued – or not – at work?
- Are there any ways in which you could try to tackle some of the hygiene factors that are negatively affecting your work experience? If so, how could you do this?
- If you have direct influence over company culture, what small changes could be made immediately to help your employees feel more valued?

Working in alignment with your values is a critical part of burnout recovery, and something we'll touch on further in Part III. You can leave this work until then or, if you'd like to learn how to identify your values and engage in values-based decision-making now, please flick to p. 141.

4. Community

Building a healthy, supportive community at work – one where you feel fairly and equitably treated – goes a long way towards protecting you against burnout.

The easiest way to achieve this is to look at how your teams function and to make small but evidence-based changes in your environment that will really move the needle. The things I'm going to share are not rocket science, and might seem obvious, but you'd be surprised how a little really does go a long way!

The following are really effective when it comes to burnout prevention:

- Socialising with colleagues outside of work
- Positive social support, i.e. sharing and celebrating successes within the team
- Expressing gratitude within teams

Simple changes go a long way to help build a strong community that is protective against burnout.

Exercise 7

 Social support at work – journal prompt
Take a moment now to consider what changes could be made at work to help improve socialising or positive support.

5. Fairness

Truly effective and impactful policies to ensure that diversity, equality, inclusion and belonging are at the forefront of company culture really matter. When employees are treated fairly, everyone wins, and it's a very effective tool in protecting individuals from burnout. Yet, in some companies it feels like treating employees fairly is very difficult to achieve.
   A fair culture looks like this:

- Decision-making is transparent
- Employees have opportunities to provide feedback
- Employees have input on decisions
- Everyone is treated with respect and dignity
- Bias and discrimination are appropriately addressed

A fundamental part of creating a safe and fair working culture is being able to cultivate an environment where employees can raise concerns in a way that doesn't jeopardise their safety at work. There are lots of ways that this can be achieved, such as tackling incivility on an organisational level.

Exercise 8

Fairness at work – journal prompts

Take a moment to reflect and take stock of how fairly you are treated at work now using the following journal prompts:

- Do you feel you are treated with respect at work?
- Do you feel that correct behaviours are modelled by leaders and managers?
- Do you have opportunities to feedback concerns?
- Do you feel your concerns are listened to?
- What changes would you like to see to improve fairness at work?
- Who might be able to help you make these changes?

6. Workload

To prevent burnout, it's essential that your workload is appropriate to your skill level, knowledge base, seniority, job description, career plan and life stage. I mention life stage because so often our capacity to take on a certain workload is affected – either directly or indirectly – by what is going on outside of work. Things like bereavement or illness, for instance, might temporarily reduce your capacity for your workload, and it's important that your employer is responsive and sympathetic to this.

When it comes to workload, you want to be pleasantly stretched and challenged rather than feeling persistently overwhelmed and that you cannot manage things. Workload becomes a problem in burnout when it is either too much (in terms of volume) or not appropriate, i.e. too complex for your skillset and knowledge base.

It's OK to face increased workload temporarily. For instance, in accounting the run-up to the end of the financial year is manic, but once the new financial year starts and the deadlines lift things tend to become a little lighter and a bit of recovery is allowed. It's when the pressure is sustained over a long period of time that burnout can occur.

Productivity hacks and time-management skills will only get you so far if your workload is persistently overwhelming you. When this is the case, employers must accept responsibility for changes to how they expect staff to work, and make reasonable adjustments. In my experience, when workload is a problem in burnout, it's because it tends to be so overwhelming that individual coping strategies are not sufficient on their own.

Common Workload Problems and Solutions

Let's look at some common workload problems I see frequently in my work, and consider possible solutions for you:

Problem 1: *Your capacity for work is temporarily reduced due to other factors in your life (such as increased stress at home, i.e. new caring responsibilities or a bereavement).*

Solution: Reach out to your line manager, occupational health department or doctor (depending on what's available to you) for advice about temporary reasonable adjustments.

Problem 2: *You are constantly having to work late to meet your deadlines and finish your work.*

Solution: Assess your time-management skills – are there any improvements that can be made? If your time-management skills are not the problem, keep a record of the work that you are doing and the time it takes you before presenting it to your manager with a request for their help in making the workload more appropriate or in delegating some tasks.

Problem 3: *You are having to step up and take on roles or responsibilities outside of your job description and pay grade, either temporarily or permanently.*

Solution: Ask for additional training and/or support to allow yourself to step up well. If this is ongoing, audit the work you are doing and ask for a promotion.

Exercise 9

Raise workload issues with your employer

If you need to raise issues about your workload with your employer, work through the following steps on how to have this difficult conversation, as needed.

1. You don't necessarily have to have this conversation in person to start with (or ever, if you don't want to!). You can choose to raise the issue via email. In fact, starting off by email and having an audit trail of conversations and promises made is a helpful thing to do, regardless.

2. If you decide to meet face to face, it is worthwhile to practise what you want to say beforehand, either with others or in front of the mirror. Imagine the conversation playing out. What barriers or responses do you anticipate coming up, and how can you allow yourself to respond in a way that is respectful and calm? Ask yourself: 'What is the worst-case scenario here?' and think of a response for this. Practising will help you gain confidence too.

3. A good way to prepare to be assertive with your boss is to practise being assertive in less challenging situations first. Consider your assertiveness to be like doing weight training in the gym – you don't head to the rack to squat more than your body weight as a beginner! Start small and light and build up gently if you don't feel ready to tackle some of the bigger problems just yet. For instance, if you find talking to your boss intimidating, start by having some courageous conversations with people that you find more approachable. Alternatively, pick a problem that is small and easily fixed to raise with your boss first, such as an improvement to your workspace or schedule.

4. People in leadership or management positions are often busy with their own targets to meet, and being presented with a problem by itself to solve (i.e. your workload) might not go down

well. Offering solutions to the problem you're facing will be really helpful for them and will help set a baseline for negotiations. For example, you could suggest passing on a project to a colleague who you know is wanting more experience in that particular area, or you could suggest a weekly team meeting to assess the deadlines for the week so you can all regularly ensure that the workload distribution is fair.

5. Any change at work will need to be negotiated, and your employer might not be able to give you what you want because of wider constraints. Having an idea about what your red lines (i.e. your absolutes) are before you have a conversation is helpful. These red lines don't necessarily have to be communicated to your employer – unless, of course, you think it would be helpful to share them – but they are there to remind you of your worth and the minimum standard by which you should be treated. If your absolutes are not met, having an idea about the next steps that you want to pursue will help you to feel in control of the situation.

6. There is strength and safety in numbers. The more of you that raise the same problems, the more weight you will have in asking for the changes you need.

Burnout and Organisational Change

Before I bring this chapter to a close, I want to briefly acknowledge the elephant in the room: truly effective burnout prevention (and recovery) begins with workplace culture change, and sometimes what an individual can realistically change is limited.

For those of us who have already burned out, recovery is focused on making changes at work in order to tackle the root cause of our stress, i.e. to reduce the risk of burnout happening again. If you think about it, the same workplace culture that caused burnout is not going to necessarily be conducive to recovery from burnout, or the right environment for avoiding burnout in the future, unless changes are made.

Leaders of organisations and businesses where a burnout culture is tolerated and perpetuated must take responsibility for leading changes from the top down. But the sad truth is that this isn't going to happen in every workplace with burnout culture. Even if positive change is happening in your workplace, it might not be happening quickly enough for you.

As we'll see in Part III, successful burnout recovery doesn't always require drastic moves such as leaving your job, but there does come a point where – if the workplace factors that caused your burnout are so entrenched – you might need to consider this as an option. You need to decide if your working environment is right for you.

During my own burnout, I realised that the workplace that burned me out was not able to make, nor sustain, the changes needed for me to recover and stay well. So, I made the decision to leave, and I do not regret it. Burnout is a problem that happens as a result of the environment that you're in, and if you can't change the environment enough, put a plan together and get out as quickly as you can.

Exercise 10

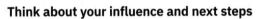

Think about your influence and next steps

Once you have completed all the exercises outlined in this chapter, ask yourself: do you think you have enough influence to be able to bring about the changes that you need to either prevent your stress levels getting worse or to recover from burnout (if this is currently where you're at)?

If you think you do have enough influence, now is the perfect opportunity to reflect on your next steps, i.e. who to approach or what help you might need to allow you to make sufficient changes. (Skip to p. 181 to read my advice on how to advocate for yourself in burnout, which will be really helpful for you at this point!)

If you don't think you have enough influence, you might want to think about exploring your career options. (The section on p. 151 about exploring work options in burnout recovery is the ideal next step for you, and this is just as relevant for those of you who are focused on burnout prevention right now too, i.e. those who are stressed at work but not burned out yet!)

Chapter 2 Takeaways

- The six workplace factors that cause burnout are: control, reward, values, community, fairness and workload. All you need is one of these factors to be mismatched to risk burnout.
- Having an idea of the workplace factors that are directly impacting on your stress levels is essential for knowing where to specifically target either your burnout prevention or burnout recovery efforts.
- Sometimes you will have sufficient influence to make enough changes at work to either prevent a burnout or recover from one. But, for some, this influence will not be enough. While you don't necessarily need to make drastic changes, if organisational change just isn't happening – or if it isn't happening fast enough – you will need to consider your career options.

3

Individual factors that cause burnout

We have talked about the workplace factors that cause burnout, but it's important to be aware that each of us has our own individual risk factors for burnout, too. These factors make us either more or less predisposed to developing burnout. This is why, as discussed previously, a group of people subjected to the same stress will not all react in the same way – some will burn out and others will not.

Getting a sense of your own individual risk factors to burnout is helpful, and that's what we'll be working through in this chapter. If you work in a high-stress job but aren't burned out yet, then knowing *how* you are predisposed to burnout means you can be proactive about managing your risk factors to avoid it. Or, if you feel that you are already burned out, understanding the risk factors that fuelled your burnout will help you to target your recovery efforts effectively and precisely.

As well as individual risk factors, there are also certain demographics in society that have shown to be more at risk of developing burnout too, and we'll touch on these at the end of this chapter. Knowing if you are in a higher risk group means you can again be proactive about burnout prevention or more knowledgeable and targeted about your burnout recovery, depending on your current circumstances. Similarly, if you are an employer, then being aware of these higher risk groups will mean you then know to offer appropriate and targeted supportive measures.

As you read through this section, take note of any individual risk factors or groups that you identify with – I'll be providing you with strategies and next steps for managing them, too.

When it comes to burnout, individual risk factors are typically linked to your personality type, past events and/or any mental health problems (either that you're facing now or that you've experienced in the past).

We can categorise the nine main individual risk factors as follows:

1. Imposter syndrome
2. Perfectionism
3. People pleasing
4. Personality type
5. Your childhood
6. Trauma in adulthood
7. Pre-existing mental health problems
8. Coping skills
9. Neurodiversity

As a reminder, if you find that you have a high individual risk factor for burnout, this does not mean that you should blame yourself if you do experience burnout. It also certainly does not mean that you are *solely* responsible for making changes in the workplace or in how you manage your personal risk factors in the workplace, either. It's not your fault.

When I first came across these risk factors, I identified so hard with so many of them. For example I'm a 'people pleaser' and 'perfectionist' by nature, which meant I allowed my workplace boundaries to be crossed repeatedly and this unfortunately contributed to my burnout. I had always been seen as a 'coper' throughout my time at medical school and postgraduate training, but my coping strategies were just not robust enough when put under sustained pressure. (The ultimate irony of burnout is that it often occurs in people who have a strong work ethic, who feel emotionally invested in their work, and who struggle to establish boundaries between work and personal life, as we'll soon discover...)

Having the knowledge now that I am a high-risk individual when it comes to burnout has helped me manage my stress better and stay well. So, let's see if you can relate to any of the below...

1. Imposter Syndrome

If you are someone who identifies with worrying that you are a fraud and not worthy of the success that you've achieved, then you might have imposter syndrome. This is when high-achieving individuals worry that they are not worthy of success and have a persistent belief in their lack of intelligence, skills or competence – despite objective evidence to the contrary. It also means that you are less likely to engage with self-care and are more likely to suffer from emotional exhaustion (which is the first step on the path to burnout syndrome, as we learned on p. 19). Up to 70 per cent of people experience some degree of imposter syndrome at some point in their lives, and as it's directly linked to burnout and poor mental health it's important to tackle it head on.

Signs of Imposter Syndrome

Imposter syndrome can show up in a variety of ways, including:

- **Overworking** – to compensate for perceived inadequacies.
- **Procrastinating and avoidance** – because you are worried about failure.
- **Downplaying your knowledge, abilities or skills** – and trying to get as many certifications and diplomas as possible to showcase your value to others, as you feel you are not enough.
- **Perfectionism** – as you look over every single detail and check your emails, papers and exams thousands of times to ensure they're perfect. (Of course, you never feel they actually are perfect!) You feel the pressure to perform at your best in every

circumstance, and when you don't, you feel incompetent and anxious.

- **Seeking our mentors and constant feedback** – that is, external validation of your performance. You want to find ways to improve until you feel like you're enough, but you never achieve this.
- **Comparing yourself to others constantly** – questioning why others got a promotion, more money or a better qualification than you. You want to be the best. Always.
- **Lacking confidence** – when showing your accomplishments, speaking up or contributing. You're afraid of being seen as silly or ignorant.

Exercise 11

Imposter syndrome – journal prompts
If you identify with having imposter syndrome, take a moment to consider:

- How does your imposter show up for you?
- What does your imposter syndrome make you think, do and miss out on?

Debunking Imposter Syndrome Myths

There are numerous myths surrounding imposter syndrome. Let's tackle some of these now, so we can get a clearer sense of what it actually is.

Myth 1: 'Imposter syndrome is your fault'

People with imposter syndrome actually develop it due to a complex interplay of factors, including their background, upbringing, experiences and environment. The common factor is often a seed of unworthiness that was planted in early life, which was then triggered into imposter syndrome as an adult by circumstances and environmental factors. For instance, there are certain jobs that train for perfection (such as surgery), and imposter syndrome is fuelled intensely under these conditions.

Myth 2: 'Confident people don't get imposter syndrome'

Imposter syndrome tends to affect people who are smart and capable. While they might appear confident externally, they may be struggling internally. You might be surprised to hear that seemingly confident individuals, such as Michelle Obama, have admitted to having imposter syndrome.

Myth 3: 'Imposter syndrome can be eased by success'

The majority of people with imposter syndrome are talented and have a long list of achievements. New or continued success does not unfortunately provide relief for the imposter syndrome sufferer. You cannot just work harder to overcome imposter syndrome.

For me, post-burnout, the biggest surprise was coming to terms with the fact that working hard and having academic and professional success was never going to satisfy my inner imposter. No matter what I achieved, I was never satisfied or thought I was worthy of my success. Instead, tackling my imposter syndrome has meant delving into the root causes of it and changing my patterns of thinking.

Myth 4: 'Imposter syndrome can be solved by removing yourself from a toxic work environment'

While certain environments are triggering, habitual self-sabotage caused by imposter syndrome means that your brain starts to believe your repetitive thoughts of negativity. Therefore removal from the triggering environment will unfortunately not be sufficient by itself to change ingrained patterns of thinking within yourself.

Myth 5: 'Imposter syndrome can be solved by awareness and positive thinking'

If only it were that easy! Overcoming imposter syndrome requires the use of psychological techniques to change ingrained patterns of thinking and to improve self-worth. While this is hard work and it may take time, it can be done!

How to Manage your Imposter Syndrome

I once attended a medical leadership conference where, during a talk on imposter syndrome, we were told: 'Girls, imposter syndrome is a construct of the patriarchy, just ignore it!' I have never forgotten this statement, mostly because it's wrong (men are affected by imposter syndrome just as much as women), but also because if it were that easy to ignore, then the 70 per cent of people who are affected by imposter syndrome in their professional lives would simply move on. But we know this isn't the case. We also know that imposter syndrome causes burnout and, as already discussed, external success and achievements don't break the imposter syndrome cycle, but working on your internal self-talk will. Use the following five exercises to help you to do this. I suggest you pick one or two of these exercises to try consistently for a couple of weeks when your imposter syndrome is playing up.

Exercise 12

Be your own cheerleader
Our own internal self-talk can be brutally harsh in imposter syndrome. This exercise helps you to learn some positive self-talk.

Think of a loved one who you care for deeply and are always on side with. Now imagine they are sat in front of you, telling you that they are experiencing exactly what you're experiencing with your imposter syndrome.

What would you say to them to make them feel better? Remember, you are totally on their side and have their back! Write down the statements you'd tell them.

Now, read those statements back to yourself and see how you feel. Do this whenever you experience harsh internal self-talk.

Exercise 13

Keep an evidence diary

Keeping an evidence diary where you write down details of all your achievements, positive feedback and compliments can be really helpful at times when your inner imposter is wild!

I keep mine electronically in my e-portfolio. I know others that keep a file on their computer, or mailbox in their emails. You could use a note-taking app too. However you do it, remember to look at it regularly when you need a little boost.

Exercise 14

Break the cycle of rumination

This exercise helps you to actively move from rumination to positive self-reflection.

After noticing any difficult or unwanted emotion (such as guilt or shame), ask yourself 'why' questions. For instance, say you had a difficult conversation with a colleague that left you feeling upset, you could ask yourself, 'Why was I triggered by the comment they made?' Really dig into the root cause of your discomfort.

Once you have identified this, plan out the action steps necessary for you to move forward and beyond this event (we will discuss SMARTR goals later, *see* p. 174). This way you're not necessarily tackling your thoughts of being an imposter, but you *are* actively changing your behaviour.

Exercise 15

'I am feeling' statements

Start using 'I am feeling' statements instead of 'I am' statements when you experience imposter syndrome.

For example, instead of your mind saying, 'I am a fraud', say to yourself 'I am *feeling* like a fraud'. You could even go one step further and start saying to yourself, 'I am *noticing* that I am feeling like a fraud.' Play with this sentence structure and observe how you feel.

This exercise will stop the emotion you're feeling from becoming your identity, as is so often experienced in imposter syndrome.

Exercise 16

Graded exposure

This exercise is for all the perfectionist imposters out there! This one always gets a sharp intake of breath and a bit of metaphorical pearl clutching in the webinars and lectures I do, because it can be quite confronting for perfectionists.

Graded exposure asks you to deliberately make a small, intentional mistake that means something you share is not perfect. The suggested way to start this is to make a deliberate typo in an email or message, and send it anyway. I would not suggest doing this in anything where it really matters (you might not be able to do this with important clients, for instance), but you might be able to do it in a WhatsApp message to your friend when you're arranging to meet them for dinner.

The idea is to make a small imperfect error and then to see what happens. You'll see that the world doesn't implode or stop turning, and that it's OK to not be perfect. Over time, you will be able to allow yourself to make bigger 'mistakes' and your perfectionist imposter will become easier to manage.

2. Perfectionism

Perfectionism – the tendency to set excessively high standards for oneself and to engage in overly self-critical thoughts and behaviours – is the second individual high-risk factor that directly feeds into burnout.

For perfectionists, anything less than 'perfect' means failure. Even if you are successful, the success is often disregarded. As a perfectionist, if you cannot disregard your success then your focus will normally shift to questioning how you will be able to keep up with it. You see, with perfectionism you end up focusing on the unattainable place you want to get to, rather than the process and the learning of the journey. When you aim for the unattainable, you always fall short. Over time, perfectionism pushes people into avoidance or overwork.

The Perfectionist Cycle

The perfectionist cycle is shown in the image below. You start in the top left-hand corner with the feeling that you don't know what you're doing, which then leads to discomfort and anxiety. You go around the cycle (anti-clockwise) and ultimately end up succeeding. However, once you get to success, your perfectionism immediately means that it's discounted, and the cycle begins again. If you recognise this cycle, you are a fellow perfectionist!

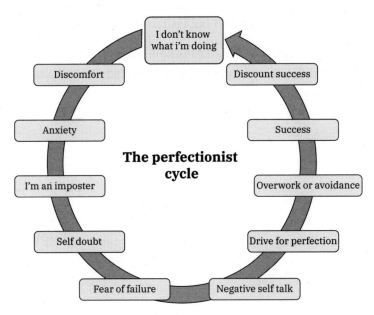

Being a perfectionist contributes to the development of burnout through:

1. **Prompting you to take on too much work** – believing that you are the only one that can complete it to your high standards. Over time, this leads to excessive workload and burnout.

2. **Experiencing a lack of satisfaction** – success does not placate the perfectionist. Instead, perfectionists are never satisfied with their work, leading to poor motivation and a sense of futility. Perfectionism can directly cause reduced job satisfaction and burnout.

3. **Increasing your 'emotional exhaustion'** – one of the three components of burnout syndrome, as discussed on p. 19. Perfectionists tend to feel the stress of relentlessly striving for perfectionism and this – combined with their fear of failure – leads to exhaustion.

So, tackling perfectionism is really key for both burnout prevention and recovery.

How to Manage your Perfectionism

Perfectionism and people pleasing (as we'll discuss opposite) can broadly be managed in the same way, so I have put the advice on how to start to manage perfectionism and people pleasing together on p. 69. Feel free to skip to there now if you'd like this information immediately.

Exercise 17

Perfectionism – journal prompts

If you identify with the perfectionist cycle (*see* p. 65), ask yourself the following questions:

- Can you think when the perfectionist cycle might have started for you?
- What events caused your perfectionism to develop?
- How does perfectionism show up for you in your daily life?
- What good has perfectionism brought you?
- How has perfectionism held you back?

3. People Pleasing

The next individual risk factor for burnout is people pleasing. People pleasing presents itself as the tendency to prioritise other people's needs, wants and desires over our own. It tends to arise in childhood and is often – but not always – secondary to strict parenting, neglect, violence, or high expectations of behaviour and achievement placed on you as a child. Here, a child may learn to suppress their wants and needs in order to keep the adults in their lives happy. What starts as an internal mechanism can be carried by the child into adulthood and develop into people pleasing.

Once established as a habit, people pleasing can lead to:

* Harsh self-criticism
* Feelings of unworthiness
* Experiential avoidance
* Disconnection with values
* Feelings of low self-worth, as you become so used to putting other people before you
* Burnout

There are six key characteristics of a people pleaser:

1. **A feeling of 'I'm not good enough'** – this is the deep sense of low self-worth, poor self-esteem and harsh self-judgement that is central to people-pleasing behaviours, as the people pleaser is so used to thinking of everyone else before themselves.
2. **Rigid rules** – people pleasers apply internal pressure and anxiety to follow self-imposed, rigid rules. For example, thinking: 'I must', 'I have to' or 'other people's needs come first'.
3. **Fear about breaking these self-imposed and rigid rules** – worrying what others would think of them.
4. **Strong experiential avoidance** – people pleasers try to escape and avoid difficult emotions. They may avoid doing things that are difficult, such as saying no to something they think they don't

want to do (for fear of letting others down). By doing this, they might miss out on things that they'd actually find fun or fulfilling because they are using their time to prioritise the needs of others over themselves. Doing this continuously means they are missing out on things that would make them happy.

5. **Lack of awareness of basic personal rights and boundaries** – people pleasers often lose sight of the fact that they have the right to be treated fairly and respectfully, and in the same way that they treat others. This may lead to people pleasers accepting poor behaviour from others.

6. **Anxiety** – people pleasing tends to be accompanied by anxiety, which unfortunately then becomes the fuel for more people pleasing (because the people pleaser assumes this will be the solution to the anxiety). One of the problems with people pleasing is that it is often used to provide temporary relief from anxiety, and sometimes the behaviour is even values congruent – as the behaviours typically centre around caring and loving. However, in the long run, people pleasing can cause more anxiety and poor mental well-being, and continuing with people pleasing can becoming exhausting, which leads to burnout.

Ultimately, those who have a strong desire to please others may take on too much work or have a hard time saying no to requests from colleagues, which can lead to burnout due to excessive workload and emotional exhaustion.

Exercise 18

 People pleasing – journal prompts
Reflect on your people pleasing and write down some notes for the following questions:

- Do you identify with being a people pleaser?
- What do you think is the root cause of your people pleasing (for example, childhood events, low self-esteem or a difficulty understanding social interactions due to neurodivergence)?

- How has people pleasing helped you?
- How has it negatively affected you?

How to Manage Perfectionism and People Pleasing

People pleasing and perfectionism often coexist, with perfectionism driving people-pleasing behaviour. They both share a lot of the key themes and so can be broadly tackled in the same way. Tackling perfectionism and people pleasing requires a multifaceted approach, which includes self-compassion, empathetic assertiveness and setting boundaries.

In the short term, people pleasing and perfectionism might feel good, but the long-term costs on well-being, work and relationships will be far reaching and can directly lead to burnout. Therefore, if you identify as being a perfectionist or a people pleaser, it's essential to work on mitigating these traits using the following pointers.

Know Your Personal Rights

As a people pleaser, it can be difficult to both be aware of and to genuinely believe that your personal rights matter. But if you don't recognise that your personal rights are important, you'll never have the confidence to assert yourself or start the rest of the process to changing people-pleasing behaviour. It's that important. Use the following exercise as a starting point.

Exercise 19

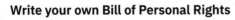

Write your own Bill of Personal Rights
Write down your own Bill of Personal Rights – either on your phone or on paper – and keep the document somewhere safe and accessible. Use the following format:

It's OK to stand up for my rights, provided I respect the rights of others as I do so; they have the same rights as I do.
I have the right to be treated fairly and respectfully.

I have the right to make my needs equally important to those of others.

I have the right to decline unreasonable requests, in a way that is fair and respectful.

I have the right to be fallible, imperfect and make mistakes.

I have the right to ask for what I want, in a way that is fair and respectful.

I have the right to honestly state my thoughts, feelings, ideas and opinions, in a way that is fair and respectful.

I have the right to ... [write your own sentence here]

When you find yourself falling into the people-pleasing cycle, read your personal rights to remind yourself of your worth.

Writing your Bill of Personal Rights may make you feel uncomfortable as a people pleaser. It is also likely to challenge some entrenched thoughts, feelings and patterns of behaviour to pursue these rights, and I imagine that there will be a lot of guilt around adopting them.

One of the keys to accepting these as your rights that you are entitled to is that it is purely about making your rights equal to those of others. It's not about you becoming the main character, or bulldozing people with unreasonable needs or requests; this is about being treated with the same respect as you disproportionately give others. It is genuinely the first step to addressing people-pleasing behaviours. If you're finding it hard to accept these rights, please take some time to think deeply about the fundamental reason(s) why you are struggling. If these reasons are very big, you might benefit from having some therapy to unpick things in a deep but safe way.

Learn to Say No

Declining requests and saying no is difficult for people pleasers. A good place to start is to give a softener to begin your rejection. Saying something along the lines of, 'I'd love to help you but...' and then giving your reasons will help to soften the blow and mean the other person is more likely to accept your boundary. Build up to saying no – start with small situations where the consequences are fewer, and then gradually challenge yourself to be assertive in more challenging scenarios.

Give Honest Feedback, Opinions and Feelings

When making requests or giving honest opinions, feelings and feedback, it's important to give 'I' statements before following up with an assertive request for behaviour changes. Using an 'I' statement, as opposed to a 'you' statement, minimises conflict. For example, say things like, 'I feel X when you do Y', or 'I feel X when you do Y because Z'.

Break Your Own Rules

This is a hard one for people pleasers and perfectionists, but challenge yourself to break one of your self-imposed rules and do something different to what your mind is telling you. Start simple and safe and then begin breaking your own rules in more challenging ways, making sure any rule breaking you do is in line with your values and values-based goals. Over time, you can really start to work on the rules that are having the most negative impact in your life.

Here are some ideas on how you can work on breaking your self-imposed rules to tackle the problem that is most appropriate to you:

- **For difficulty in declining unreasonable requests** – practise assertively declining requests.
- **For avoiding feedback (for fear it could be negative)** – practise actively asking for feedback and constructive criticism.
- **For risk aversion** – practise taking small but sensible risks then gradually increase the risk factor.
- **For indecisiveness (fear of making the 'wrong' decision and upsetting others)** – set a significantly shorter-than-usual time limit for a decision to be made – and stick to it.
- **For excessive workload (taking too much on board; setting unrealistic deadlines)** – practise assertively declining extra work and/or assertively setting realistic timelines.

- **For fear of making mistakes** – practise deliberately making mistakes (where the real-life consequence is minimal).
- **For avoidance of asking for help** – practise deliberately asking for help or delegating.
- **For setting unrealistic goals** – practise setting SMARTR goals (*see* p. 174) and sticking to them.

Set Realistic Goals

Perfectionists are likely to find it difficult to set achievable goals, at least initially. Instead of making your goals achievable, try to make them *adaptive*. This means ensuring that your goals are achievable, given your current capacity and resources. It's essentially asking if your goals are compassionate, sympathetic and appropriate for you in your current circumstances and frame of mind.

4. Personality Types

Your personality type might very well put you at increased risk of burnout. This is interesting because as a type-A, highly empathetic and introverted person (I'm an INTJ [Introvert/Intuitive/Thinking/Judging], in case you want to know!), I previously had no idea that my personality primed me for burnout, but that's exactly what it did. Let's run through the key factors here so you can know the personality traits that put you at high risk.

People with type-A personalities tend to be highly ambitious, competitive and driven, which can lead them to take on too many responsibilities and work longer hours than necessary. This can lead to burnout due to the constant pressure to achieve and exceed goals.

People who have a high level of empathy and compassion may take on too much emotional labour, resulting in burnout due to the emotional exhaustion of constantly supporting others.

Extroversion appears to be protective against burnout, while introverts tend to be more at risk. Introverts tend to have a lower threshold for external stimulation and may become overstimulated in noisy or busy environments. This can be especially draining for introverts who work in highly social or extroverted fields, such as sales or customer service, where extrovert demands are placed on them. Constant interaction with people can be exhausting for introverts and lead to burnout if they don't have enough alone time to recharge.

Introverts instead may find more energy and fulfilment in solitary or quiet activities, such as reading or working independently. If their work allows for a more independent and introspective environment, introverts may be less likely to experience burnout.

Introverts who work in high-demand jobs are more likely to experience burnout than extroverts in the same type of job. This may be because introverts are less likely to seek social support or engage in social coping strategies, which can protect against burnout. People who are extroverted tend to be more protected from emotional exhaustion and burnout through the interpersonal bonds they create and their typically positive outlook at work.

The key point here in determining whether an introvert is more at risk of burnout or not is the type of job that is being done. I am highly introverted and I now recognise that working in a medical job that requires me to be extroverted, without adequate downtime to recharge my energy, put me at increased risk of burnout. Sitting in a clinic, seeing up to 50 patients a day, with multiple interruptions from colleagues... that's painful for an introvert without proper breaks in place! Conversely, the work I do on social media has been OK as an introvert, mainly because I can choose how and when to interact with people.

Exercise 20

 Your personality type – journal prompts
Take a moment to consider your personality type, and how it affects your risk of burnout:

* Do you identify with being introverted or extroverted?
* Do you work in a job that requires you to be introverted or extroverted?

How to Manage Your Personality Type

Being an introvert in an extroverted role can be a risk factor for burnout, so this is what we'll focus on here. If this is you, then looking at how you manage the needs of your personality type (whether you're at prevention or recovery stage with burnout) is crucial, particularly if you are keen to stay in your current role.

'Introvert burnout' is the term for what an introvert experiences when they engage in too much socialisation without enough time to recharge, so introverts require changes in the workplace – or changes in their life more generally – to help them prioritise moments of rest and recharge.

Here are my top tips for introverts in extroverts jobs:

1. **Focus on problem-focused coping strategies** – to help rebalance your life (*see* p. 78 on coping styles for more).
2. **Boundaries, boundaries, boundaries** – introverts have to be firm in asserting boundaries to ensure that they can make changes that help reduce the negative effects of introversion on mental well-being.

   Boundary setting at work might involve having frank conversations with others about issues, such as having 'quiet time' in your day or work week, not answering texts or emails after hours, skipping additional social time (even if it occurs virtually) and perhaps turning off your camera during video meetings.

   Boundary setting at home might involve having dedicated work hours, creating a dedicated workspace and charging your work phone out of sight. Part of effective boundary setting involves learning to say no in the right circumstances (*see* p. 182 for more on boundary setting).
3. **Prioritise exercise and movement** – outside where possible (because exposure to daylight will help with sleep quality). For introverts, online, solo or home-based options for exercise, such as running or doing body-weight exercises, might be preferable to doing group classes or joining clubs. However, having a good social support network is crucial (even for introverts), so do

consider joining a group (if you have the capacity and opportunity for meaningful downtime in other areas of your life).

4. **Find a creative outlet** – dedicating time to creative outlets such as music, art or cooking is a healthy intervention. Creativity and mastery of a skill outside of work can be a key part of recovery. For introverts, you can choose skills and hobbies that can be done solo, or where interaction can be controlled.

5. **Enlist help** – friends and family members who understand your introversion and the emotional challenges you are experiencing can be a good line of defence against taking on more. They can also provide privacy and support you in recharging.

6. **Use your rest and recovery time effectively** – *see* my advice on p. 192.

5. Your Childhood

The key things that happen in childhood that prime you for burnout are mixed messages about achievement and any Adverse Childhood Experiences (ACEs), such as abuse, neglect, trauma or bereavement.

Let's start with the impact of mixed messages about achievement. Having high parental expectations isn't necessarily a bad thing. In fact, if done well, having expectations placed on you can motivate you to achieve well and strive for success. However, if expectations are too high, inconsistent or unrealistic, or if parental love becomes conditional on success, this is when your risk of burnout as an adult increases.

The quality of your relationship with your parents also matters, as a good-quality relationship helps with emotional development and your ability to regulate stress. The combination of high expectations for achievement and low emotional support from parents confers the highest risk. This in turn directly affects your risk of burnout as an adult.

We also know that ACEs can increase your burnout risk as an adult. This is because of how they directly impact on the brain's structure and function at such a young age, before the brain is fully developed. It is thought that changes due to ACEs contribute to a dysregulated stress response as an adult, but the reasons for the increased adult burnout risk is likely to be multifactorial.

Exercise 21

 Your childhood – journal prompts
Take a moment to look back on your childhood and reflect:

- Did you feel pressure to achieve as a child?
- Do you think this was healthy or unhelpful pressure?
- Are there any childhood events that might have affected your burnout risk?

How to Manage Childhood Trauma

If you identify with any issues or events in your childhood causing you difficulties as an adult (be that through burnout or other problems, such as relationship difficulties or emotional distress), my advice is to seek expert and tailored help from a psychologist.

6. Trauma in Adulthood and PTSD

Exposure to traumatic events as an adult also puts you at increased risk of burnout. Violence – either experiencing it directly or witnessing it – accidents and natural disasters particularly confer a higher risk. This is because of how trauma affects the areas of the brain that are also affected in burnout, leading to problems with how you are able to cope with stress.

PTSD, which can develop after exposure to a traumatic event, also puts individuals at a higher risk of burnout. Interestingly, the changes that happen in the brain with PTSD are very similar to the changes that happen in burnout. Symptoms of PTSD can include:

- Hypervigilance (always being on edge, looking for danger even when you are safe)

- Avoidance
- Nightmares
- Flashbacks
- Emotional numbing

Exercise 22

 Trauma in adulthood

Take a minute to reflect: are there any traumatic events that have happened to you as an adult that might predispose you to burnout?

How to Manage Trauma in Adulthood

My advice here is to seek expert and tailored help from a psychologist. For trauma, eye movement desensitisation and reprocessing (EMDR) therapy and trauma-focused CBT are helpful to explore. EMDR helps to treat mental health problems that occur due to memories from traumatic events in your past, and works by getting you to move your eyes when you are processing these past events under instruction from a trained therapist. It might perhaps sound a little strange that eye movements can have such a profound impact, if you've not come across EMDR before, but it is incredibly effective.

7. Pre-Existing Mental Health Problems

It is probably not a surprise to learn that if you already have a mental health problem, or have experienced one in the past, you are at higher risk of burnout. In particular, the problems that are directly linked to burnout are anxiety and depression (as discussed on p. 32). People with substance misuse problems, such as alcohol or recreational drugs, are also more likely to report symptoms of burnout.

Exercise 23

Mental health – journal prompts

Think about your own mental health:

- Do you identify with having any current mental health problems?
- How are your mental health problems being managed presently?

How to Manage Pre-Existing Mental Health Problems

If you are currently experiencing symptoms of a mental health problem, please seek advice from your doctor and/or therapist, as they are best placed to advise you about how to effectively manage them.

8. Coping Styles

Even if the slide into burnout isn't consciously recognised, most people will have made attempts to feel better during that time. Some emotional coping styles (such as denial and avoidance) are associated with higher levels of burnout, while those that adopt problem-focused coping styles (such as active problem solving and seeking social support) are protected against burnout. Most people that end up in full-blown burnout will have used coping strategies to soothe how they feel about the stress, and to manage their own emotions, rather than tackling the root cause (i.e. the stressor itself); essentially, if you're able to manage your stress by tackling the root cause of it, you're much more likely to prevent burnout.

Action-focused coping styles focus on modifying the *source* of stress and solving problems, whereas emotion-centred coping styles focus on *regulating the emotional response* to stress. People that cope with stress using emotion-focused strategies generally avoid the problem by engaging in distracting activities, and seeking social support, rather than tackling the source of the stress directly.

Without doubt, emotion-focused coping styles have their place – typically in situations where you cannot control what is happening. Bereavement is an example of a situation where it's more than appropriate to use emotion-focused coping. However, in burnout recovery, it helps to move towards problem-focused coping styles, as they help to target the root cause of stress, allowing you to reduce or eliminate an issue. Problem-focused coping strategies can help some individuals feel less overwhelmed or anxious faster than other forms of stress management.

Self-efficacy is an individual's belief in their ability to perform a task or achieve a goal. Your self-efficacy can also directly affect your risk of burnout. For example, if you believe you can achieve a goal, your burnout risk is reduced. Conversely, if you don't believe you can achieve it, your burnout risk is increased. So, our mindset and the way we approach our problems can make a huge difference to our burnout risk and recovery.

I find coping styles and their link to burnout fascinating, particularly because so much of our individual burnout risks are down to things that we cannot control (such as previous exposure to trauma and how we were parented). But coping styles are absolutely things that we have agency over, which is so helpful to know!

Exercise 24

Coping styles – journal prompt
Think about your own coping style. Do you identify with using problem-focused coping strategies?

How to Manage Coping Styles

Quite often we tend to avoid dealing with the root cause of our stress. It's important to emphasise that this is completely normal – we all do it and we all think it's going to help us. Unfortunately, in burnout, it doesn't help in the long run. And in recovery, avoiding the source of our stress is also not going to help us.

What does help is changing the focus of your attempts to feel better on to the root cause, using problem-based coping. Problem-based coping is where you try to alter or manage the problem that is causing you to experience stress or emotional-based coping, which is where you think about changing or reducing the negative emotions associated with your stress.

Exercise 25

 Problem-based copings – journal prompts
Think about your biggest stressor at work right now and consider the following:

- What have you been doing to cope with this?
- Are your solutions emotion focused or problem focused?
- Can you identify a problem-based solution for this stressor?
- What are the costs and the benefits of the problem-based solution?
- What action can you take this week to manage this stressor with a problem-focused solution?

When you're in the throes of burnout, this exercise can be tricky. If you're finding it hard, I recommend going back to Exercise 4 on p. 42 to help you identify what you reasonably have control over first. Problem-focused coping is helpful when you have perceived control or a degree of control over a situation. If you feel powerless (as so often happens in burnout) remember you almost certainly have *some* control, even if you currently feel that you don't.

9. Neurodiversity

We are currently seeing a new generation – particularly of adult women – being diagnosed with Attention Deficit Hyperactivity Disorder (ADHD) and/or Autistic Spectrum Disorders (ASD). These people typically have not been diagnosed in early life because they have been able to mask their symptoms sufficiently, or perhaps because they presented in a different way to expected.

While workplaces can be difficult for folks with neurodiversity generally – diagnosed or otherwise – in both ADHD and ASD, burnout cycles are really driven by the fallout of being neurodivergent in a neurotypical world, and therefore there is a natural link between neurodiversity and burnout. Let's take a closer look at ADHD and ASD.

ADHD (Attention Deficit Hyperactivity Disorder)

ADHD is a neurodevelopmental condition that affects executive functioning, attention and impulsivity. There is evidence to suggest that ADHD is linked to burnout, and this association may be particularly relevant for women who are diagnosed later in life.

Children with ADHD tend to be very restless, fidgety and impulsive, and they often do things without thinking about them. They might struggle at school because they are not able to concentrate. However, symptoms of undiagnosed ADHD in adults are generally more subtle, as the adult brain is able to manage some of the symptoms. ADHD in adulthood might look like:

* having difficulty finishing projects once the challenging parts have been done;
* having difficulty organising tasks and getting things in order;
* forgetting appointments and obligations;
* avoiding or delaying tasks that require a lot of thought;
* needing to fidget or do something with the hands or feet when in meetings or having to sit still for long periods;
* feeling overly active and compelled to move;
* making careless mistakes when working on a tedious or repetitive task or piece of work;
* having difficulty concentrating on what people say;
* regularly losing items such as keys, wallet or phone;
* being distracted by activity and noise;
* having difficulty relaxing and unwinding;
* talking a lot in social situations, interrupting other people, finishing off other people's sentences;
* finding it hard to wait your turn in situations where this is expected or required.

You can see from the list of symptoms that people with undiagnosed ADHD are likely to struggle with some important aspects of work. In particular, difficulties with time management, organisational skills and stress management at work lead to a higher rate of burnout in those with ADHD.

I've mentioned that we are now seeing increased rates of adult women being diagnosed with ADHD, and it is thought that this group is at a higher risk of burnout due to underdiagnosis and/or misdiagnosis with mental health problems. But regardless of biological sex or gender, for people with ADHD, burnout is normally caused by unmanaged symptoms of ADHD. However, workplace stressors (particularly tight deadlines and a heavy workload requiring concentration) and unhealthy coping mechanisms (like avoidance and social withdrawal) are also factors. Masking can be very stressful, too, and certainly can factor into the development of burnout.

ASD (Autistic Spectrum Disorders)

People with ASD may be more prone to experiencing burnout due to the unique challenges they face in the workplace and in other areas of life. Problems might include sensory overload, difficulty with social interaction and challenges with executive functioning, which can lead to increased stress and anxiety in demanding environments. An individual with ASD may struggle with an open-plan office, for example, due to sensory overload or difficulty filtering out distracting background noise.

Alternatively, people with ASD may have difficulty with the social expectations of office culture, such as small talk and non-verbal communication, which can lead to feelings of isolation and anxiety. These challenges may make it harder for individuals with ASD to cope with the demands of their job and manage their workload effectively.

Autistic burnout is conceptualised as resulting from chronic life stress and a mismatch of expectations and abilities without adequate support. It is characterised by exhaustion, loss of function and reduced tolerance to stimulus. Autistic burnout typically starts during puberty and then can flare again during life transitions or changes, but it can happen at any age.

Exercise 26

Neurodivergence – journal prompts
Consider the following:

- Do you have a diagnosis of neurodivergence?
- If yes, how has your diagnosis impacted on how you cope with stress?
- What mechanisms do you have in place to help you manage your stress?
- Do you recognise some of the features of neurodivergence and wonder if you might have a missed or delayed diagnosis?
- If so, would pursuing a diagnosis help you?

How to Manage ADHD Burnout and Neurodiversity

ADHD is directly linked to burnout, and there has been a lot of scientific work done to prove this. However, quite shockingly, there is very little work done on how to successfully manage burnout in ADHD (just three studies known to me at the time of writing!). The difficulty with this lack of scientific work and evidence-based advice means that when there is an information vacuum, it gets filled with advice that doesn't necessarily work or isn't always helpful. While I know a lot about burnout, I'm not an expert on ADHD myself. Therefore, I've consulted with doctors and neuroscientists so that I could put together the very best advice for you here if you have ADHD burnout.

ADHD burnout is a state of stress and exhaustion that can develop when people are struggling with the stress of unmanaged ADHD symptoms for a long period of time. It follows a slightly different pattern to burnout in those that are neurotypical. For those that are neurotypical, there tends to be a build-up of symptoms and stressors before hitting burnout, and while you might find that recovery is not necessarily linear and you might slide back into burnout, the recovery processes are perhaps a little clearer without the overlay of ADHD.

ADHD also tends to cause more cyclical burnout, as ADHD symptoms make it hard to commit and follow through on work tasks. This then leads to an accumulation of stress, unhealthy coping techniques (such as avoidance, procrastination and self-medication) then withdrawal (quitting, giving up on tasks and withdrawing socially), before going back to feeling overwhelmed and stressed. People with ADHD take significantly more stress-related days off sick than those that do not have ADHD.

Work stressors are a factor in the ADHD burnout cycle, but fundamentally the cycle is driven by the ADHD itself. Therefore, the recovery processes discussed in the rest of this book will not be enough to break the ADHD burnout cycle alone. There are some extra things to be aware of that will need your attention in order to successfully break the cycle of ADHD burnout.

Managing your ADHD symptoms will form a key part of the recovery process. Unmanaged, the symptoms of ADHD can make it very difficult to focus, sit still and complete tasks on time. Regardless of whether you manage this with medication, therapy or changes to your routine or work habits, it's important to reduce the negative impact of these symptoms on your work to help manage burnout.

Procrastination and avoidance can also factor into ADHD burnout, because these cause stress by creating a backlog of tasks. Impulsivity can lead to not finishing work tasks and taking on too much. Taking on too many responsibilities and tasks is a common pitfall of people with ADHD, who tend to have a lot of energy, motivation and optimism about how much they can do. Unfortunately, they may not be realistic with themselves or others about how much they can do or how quickly they can accomplish their goals.

ADHD masking can also be exhausting. Not only does it contribute to ADHD burnout directly in itself, it can also affect relationships and expectations from employers and co-workers.

How to Break the Cycle of ADHD Burnout

Dr Zoe Watson, GP and ADHD coach, has three core principles that underpin her ADHD coaching. She says,

Everyone with ADHD is different. There's no one-size-fits-all like everything in life and medicine. The biggest thing is learning self-acceptance and self-kindness because I think some ADHD coaches will teach people strategies that are based on what neurotypical people use as coping strategies. But, those strategies never work, as neurodivergent brains are literally wired differently. So, if you try and teach someone with ADHD coping strategies, like using a planner, it's just not going to work, because the brain is just not going to go there. A lot of what I do initially is about exploring the things that they're finding difficult, and then allowing them space to speak kindly to themselves, and to accept their neurodivergence.

Here I combine Dr Zoe's advice with my own on how best to break the ADHD burnout cycle:

1. **Access specialist support from an ADHD-trained therapist (CBT or DBT) or coach**, if you can. Dialectical behaviour therapy (DBT) is a type of talking therapy based on CBT. It's designed to be particularly helpful for people who feel emotions very intensely. DBT and CBT can help with training in organisation, planning and time management; problem-solving skills; techniques for reducing distraction and increasing attention span; and cognitive restructuring, particularly around situations that cause distress. It's pretty much everything you need to know to successfully break the ADHD burnout cycle!

   Of note, inattention is a stronger predictor of burnout than hyperactivity, so putting measures in place to help with focus in particular will really help. However, while CBT is recommended to help control ADHD symptoms, not everyone with ADHD feels it is helpful for them, so if this is you then you're certainly not alone. Read on to find out some more ways of breaking the ADHD burnout cycle.

2. **Medication might be helpful** for controlling symptoms and minimising their impact on your burnout risk. You don't need to take medication every day if you don't want or need to – most people take medication on work, university or school days when they need to focus or quieten down their brains. Of course, any decision to take medication must be based on understanding the risks and benefits, so please speak to your doctor if you think this would be helpful for you.

3. **Understanding your neurodivergent brain** is a key first step to comprehending why you find certain aspects of life and work difficult. Knowledge is empowerment!

4. **Get help to learn self-compassion and self-acceptance skills.** Dr Zoe advises:

> *Generally, once women come to me having lived usually 30 or 40 years of having a neurodivergent brain and trying to exist in a neurotypical society, they are carrying a whole heap of shame. They've been told repeatedly throughout their life that they're lazy, they're not good enough, that they're stupid. They absorb all of that and they believe it.*

Learning to let go of all of this lightens the load and enables you to move on with successfully tackling the factors that are fuelling your ADHD burnout.

5. **Learning to talk openly about yourself as a neurodivergent person** is helpful for breaking the burnout cycle. Dr Zoe explains:

> *A lot of times they'll be hiding [their neurodivergence] from their employer because they're scared that if they share that they are a person with ADHD, they're going to be not good enough to do the job they're already doing. So, we will talk about strategies and ways that they can start talking to their employers.*

She stresses that, under the Disability Inclusion Act in the UK, you have additional workplace rights and funding if you have ADHD.

6. **Unmask your ADHD and use your support networks.** Masking is exhausting. Let the mask drop. Be honest about your ADHD with yourself and the people around you, and let them help you! It'll feel a much lighter burden to carry when you do this.

   This is difficult for those that are as yet undiagnosed – we know that there are currently a large number of adults that are being diagnosed with ADHD in adulthood, being as they were able to successfully mask their symptoms as a child, so if this is you do speak to your doctor about what routes to diagnosis are available.

7. **Request appropriate reasonable adjustments from your employer**, in order to help ease the impact of your ADHD symptoms on your work life and subsequent stress levels. Dr Zoe says:

   Open-plan offices are the absolute bane of neurodivergent people's existence because of the sensory overwhelm. They are absolutely horrific for productivity and for burnout. Ideally, you would have the option of having your own office, but if you can't do that, you can have noise-cancelling headphones. You can also create a decompression room where they can go when they're struggling and need to release.

   There are many things your employer can do to help you at work.

8. **Practice mindfulness.** Regular mindfulness exercises reduce inattentiveness, hyperactivity and impulsivity in people with ADHD. Mindfulness also has a secondary benefit in reducing stress and preventing burnout. If meditating isn't your thing, then doing flow/meditative activities such as yoga and Tai Chi are just as beneficial.

Managing Other Forms of Neurodiversity

There are many other forms of neurodiversity that can factor into your experience of workplace stress and/or affect your ability to manage your stress well, beyond ADHD and ASD. My advice for those who identify with any of this is to reach out for expert support, particularly in the workplace, so that you can have reasonable adjustments made to help reduce your burnout risk.

For other forms of neurodiversity, successfully tackling burnout also means learning effective strategies to manage the thoughts, feelings and behaviours caused by the neurodivergence that then put you at risk of burnout. Please seek expert advice from your doctor or specialist nurse/ therapist if this is you.

Demographics at Risk of Burnout

It's not just personality traits that put you at high risk of burnout; it's also been proven that certain demographics in society are more vulnerable to burnout. So, if you belong to any of the groups listed here, you'll be more susceptible to burnout:

- **Professionals in high-stress occupations:** The highest risk jobs for burnout are healthcare, law, finance, technology, teaching and social workers. Entrepreneurs and business owners also have a higher risk.
- **Parents and caregivers:** Anyone who cares for others – even if the work is unpaid – is at risk of burnout. Limited time, lack of support and guilt can prevent this demographic from seeking help, which can put them at higher risk.
- **Students:** The difficulties associated with academic pressure, deadlines, competition, debt and parental expectations impact directly on burnout risk.
- **Marginalised communities:** Some ethnic minorities, LGBTQIA+ individuals and people with disabilities may face unique stressors, which contribute to burnout. This vulnerability to burnout is compounded by the effects of microaggressions, discrimination,

social and health inequalities and additional barriers to accessing help that people in marginalised communities face.

- **Younger adults:** Gen Z – the most stressed age group in the workplace – are more at risk of burnout compared to Gen X. This is thought to be because changes to working practices and working culture after the pandemic disproportionately affected this particular generation.

I want to make the point here that just because you might identify as having high individual risk factors or be part of a high-risk demographic, burnout doesn't happen without environmental factors too, i.e. the workplace factors we discussed in Chapter 2. Knowing the individual risk factors for burnout goes some way to explaining why you can take a group of professionals and subject them to the same stresses at work, and some people will burn out and others won't. Some of us are primed for it, others are not.

Equally, when it comes to burnout recovery you must tackle some of your own individual risk factors for burnout, but we also know that any intervention that focuses solely on the individual (such as mindfulness techniques) alone will not be sufficient. Burnout requires an approach that tackles your risk factors alongside changes at work (as we'll be exploring in more detail in Part III).

Burnout and Women

I have long carried a view that burnout – despite its official WHO definition as a workplace problem (*see* p. 19) – occurs at the intersection between the demands of work and other concurrent stressors and demands in your life. If you're a woman, you're more likely to shoulder these increased demands outside of work.

According to a survey in the US, mothers are 28 per cent more likely than fathers to burn out. There was an estimate of over 2 million additional cases of burnout among working mothers during the 2020 pandemic due to the unequal demands of home and work. This is not to say that men don't burn out, because they do, but women as a demographic are more at risk.

Furthermore, it's Black, Asian and Latina mothers that suffer the highest levels of burnout in the US. This makes a lot of sense to me. A Black mother in her thirties will have a very different experience at work to that of a white man in his fifties in the same company, and these experiences are not solely down to any differing levels of seniority between them. The Black woman might well be subject to microaggressions, unconscious bias and possibly discrimination, for example, in addition to all of the logistical and financial penalties that being a working mother brings, such as juggling childcare. The woman's experience of the workplace in this example is therefore very likely to be more stressful than the experience of someone who is not from Black, Asian or Latina communities. When we factor in the already pre-existing additional pressures of being a woman and a mother (including the gender pay gap, *see* p. 44), you can really appreciate why women who are Black, Asian or Latina are more at risk of burnout. Recognition and validation of the different experiences of women at work is really important for effective burnout prevention and recovery.

The Mental Load

In cis-heterosexual relationships, women do more of the household chores compared to men, even when both spouses work full-time jobs, and this gap gets bigger when a couple has children. But it's not just the physical load that women take on disproportionately.

Outside of professional work, the mental load of keeping a family and/or household running commonly falls to women. For example, women are often primarily responsible for keeping household routines, organising schedules, maintaining order and providing emotional support to children. This disproportionate share of the mental workload is associated with a poorer sense of well-being for women and lower levels of satisfaction with their romantic relationships.

However, the disproportionate mental load on women is in fact even more nuanced and complex than this as the mental load process can be divided into four parts. It's interesting to know that women disproportionately engage with different parts of the four-part process compared to men. The four parts of the mental load include:

1. Anticipate
2. Identify
3. Decide
4. Monitor

While both men and women participate equally on the 'decide' step, women are much more likely to handle the other steps in the process. In other words, in the majority of families women are more likely to put an item on the agenda and follow up to make sure it has been done. This is true even for household tasks assigned to the man in the household, which can be anything from DIY to the food shop!

To give an example of how this plays out, let's imagine that you are jointly considering taking on a kitchen renovation in the home. 'Anticipate' means to anticipate any needs. For a kitchen renovation, this might mean looking at the space and how best to use it for the needs of the family. 'Identify' means assessing the options available. This might involve comparing options online or offline. For a kitchen, this might mean looking at Pinterest or Instagram for some design inspiration and then going to look at showroom kitchens. 'Decide' means to decide from the different options that are available, and 'Monitor' would mean monitoring the process and ensuring that you get the result you wanted, i.e. making sure that the renovation runs smoothly, right from purchasing the items to supervising the kitchen fitters. In this example, both parties will join in with deciding on a kitchen from the options available, but the woman is far more likely to do all of the other tasks of the mental load. What this means in practice is that women don't just disproportionally take on more of the mental load, they also take on the most draining bits. No wonder women – mothers particularly – are knackered, and burning out hard and fast.

Women's Health

The increased burnout risk on women can also be linked to health problems and life events. This can include (but is not limited to): period problems, menopause, fertility problems, pregnancy and post-partum. All of these things take a huge toll on a woman's emotional well-being and capacity to deal with work stress. For instance, the menstrual cycle (a monthly and entirely normal bodily event for 50 per cent of the population) has been demonstrated to have a moderate to severe impact on workplace productivity and increased absenteeism rates.

Midwife and author Leah Hazard (46) describes the convergence of workplace factors, perimenopause and bereavement in the development of her burnout:

I had been working as a midwife for nine years at the time of my burnout in 2020. This was already an incredibly challenging role and, as a midwife predominantly based in the maternity triage unit, I was very much at the frontline of a service well past breaking point. The workload was extreme, complex and relentless.

I would say that my burnout came to a crisis point in the August of that year, but it had been an awful year from the start. My father had a prolonged illness and died in April. I had been having some pretty acute health problems of my own, and then in June I caught Covid for the first time from an unmasked patient. I was extremely unwell and took about six weeks to return to work, throwing myself straight back into night shifts, followed quickly by days.

I began to feel numb, dissociated and anxious, but on a particularly busy and understaffed day at work I had a massive panic attack that actually felt like I was about to have a stroke. Being in hospital, I was able to check my blood pressure, which was dangerously high. I thought I might need a few days off work, but I could barely function so I ended up taking four months off. I slid into a deep depression, which in hindsight was also linked with the perimenopause.

I found it so hard to unpick the trauma I'd experienced at work from the bereavement and other health issues. I literally felt as if I lost myself, and questioned how I could ever return to work, or even to that building.

Chapter 3 Takeaways

- The predisposing risk factors to burnout are: imposter syndrome, perfectionism, people pleasing, personality type, your childhood, trauma in adulthood, pre-listing mental health problems, coping skills and neurodiversity.
- The key demographic group most at risk of burnout are mothers.
- To effectively prevent and treat burnout, you must focus on both workplace factors and individual risk factors – but this doesn't mean that the individual is at fault if they burn out.

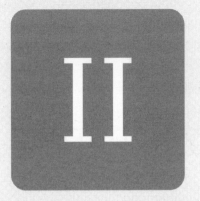

PART

II

IDENTIFYING BURNOUT

Are you burned out?

We've covered the workplace factors that cause burnout and looked at the individual risk factors that can make you more vulnerable to it. But how do you know if you're in danger of burnout or if you're actually burned out? Well, there are two resources I'd recommend, which I'll share with you in this chapter.

The first is an overview of the 'five stages of burnout' (below). I suggest you read through this and see which stage – if any – you currently identify with. I then advise that you complete the 'Burnout Assessment Tool' (*see* p. 101), which is a validated questionnaire to help individuals assess burnout and burnout risk. Together, these two tools combine to give you a fair assessment of where you stand with your current level of burnout.

Resource 1: The Five Stages of Burnout

The following five stages have been identified as the common process that most people who end up in burnout experience. It's worth noting that I don't think you necessarily have to go through each stage sequentially to end up in burnout, but I do think it is helpful to know that there is a recognised process.

This five stages of burnout model is helpful for anyone who would like to assess if they are any of the following:

- At risk of burnout
- Sliding into burnout
- Actually experiencing burnout

It's also helpful for those in recovery, as revisiting the stages and early identification of any relapse will help you to get the help you need quicker and earlier. I invite you to read through the following stages and see if you can relate to any of them now. For each stage, I give a real-life example from Kirsty Sinclair (45, teacher in a state-funded sector), who slipped through each stage of burnout through her career as a teacher (kirstyannasinclair.com).

Stage 1: Honeymoon Phase

The 'honeymoon phase' is characterised by enthusiasm for your work and is particularly relevant to new job roles or undertaking fresh work tasks and initiatives. At this stage, there are absolutely no signs of burnout. Instead, you are full of enthusiasm, commitment and joy from your work. You are very productive and take on every possible task and opportunity to perform your best. You feel creative, optimistic and full of energy. As Kirsty explains:

> *Working as a teacher initially made me feel safe and valued in society. I wanted to be the best possible teacher that I could be, and was keen to progress.*

While this stage can feel wonderful, you might take on more than you should in order to prove yourself. The risk is that if you don't prevent overworking and adopt strategies to wind down and rest regularly, you may progress to the next stage before you know it.

Stage 2: Onset of Stress

When you start noticing that some days are more stressful than others, you have progressed to the second stage of burnout. As Kirsty observes:

Reductions in education resourcing led to pressure to take on more responsibility and overlook unacceptable risks.

This stage is characterised by the following:

- lack of time for personal needs (for example, taking breaks or exercising regularly);
- seeing your family and friends less often;
- feeling that your job is the most important thing in your life.

In this stage you will likely notice the onset of physical symptoms, such as headaches or muscular pain, and psychological symptoms, such as difficulty focusing and concentrating.

Stage 3: Chronic Stress

When your stress levels become frequent and constant you are moving into this next stage: chronic stress. In this stage, your problem-solving skills and performance decrease further, and you start feeling you are out of control and powerless. Your productivity decreases, and you might find yourself procrastinating as you experience overwhelm. You may start to feel like you are not performing as well at your job, and with this comes guilt and a sense of failure. As Kirsty explains:

I put in more hours but couldn't seem to achieve much. Lots of staff continued working while unwell, and the pressure to do so was enormous. Digestive issues, insomnia, anxiety, teeth grinding, angry outbursts and social isolation were normalised in the workplace. Over-drinking and overthinking were common habits.

Chronic stress takes a toll on your mental and physical health and further intensifies the physical and psychological symptoms described in Stage 2. You may find yourself getting ill more frequently.

Additionally, you may not seem to regulate your emotions that well anymore. Issues that you could calmly manage in earlier stages now send you flying off the handle. Even small things may make you aggressive, resentful or sad. You may deny the problems and distance yourself from your colleagues and your social life. In extreme cases, to escape the negative emotions, some people may even start to self-medicate with alcohol or drugs.

Stage 4: Burnout

Kirsty reflects on her progression through the stages, approaching Stage 4, which is burnout itself, where you reach critical exhaustion levels that will make it hard to cope with work demands:

> *Dysfunction was normalised. There was a gradual increase in my stress levels over time, alongside responsibilities outside work.*

The continuous sense of failure and powerlessness eventually leads to the feeling of despair and disillusionment. You don't see 'a way out' of your circumstances and you become indifferent towards your work. Apathy is the key emotion in this stage of burnout. This sense of apathy is the 'depersonalisation' component of burnout, as described in the official WHO definition (*see* p. 19).

Burnout is a very physical experience, and this stage is also characterised by constant and disproportionate fatigue and other significant physical symptoms, such as muscle tension, headaches and stomach pains. The developed sense of self-doubt and pessimistic outlook on your job and life is pronounced.

Stage 5: Habitual Burnout

This stage is when you are unable to recover from burnout (i.e. Stage 4), and what you are experiencing becomes habitualised. Attempts to bring yourself back to normal are more challenging than ever before. Apart from affecting your career, habitual burnout may reflect in many aspects of your life, including personal relationships. You can lose joy in the hobbies that you once loved, and you may not feel like doing anything.

You may always feel sad. Not everyone with burnout has depression alongside it (*see* p. 32 for more), but if you do then it's at this stage that burnout is usually associated with clinical depression. At Stage 5, you are likely to need outside help to start to recover. The need for intervention is what characterises this particular stage, as Kirsty's story highlights:

One day I realised I couldn't go back. My breaking point was not sleeping for three consecutive nights, and a weird kind of inertia settled in; I felt as if my brain simply wouldn't work. Even simple decisions were impossible. I felt deep shock, and one day looked in the mirror and didn't recognise myself. I called a friend who was also a union rep, and on their advice I went to my GP who signed me off. I never returned.

Let's take a moment to reflect on which stage of burnout you identify with the most by completing the exercise below. The questions here reflect the fact that you might spend busier periods of work in one stage but lighter periods of work in another. That's OK. What matters is where you spend the majority of your time, and the direction of travel, i.e. are you progressively becoming more burned out?

Exercise 27

Identification of your burnout stage
Consider the following:

- When work is busy, which stage resonates most?
- When work is easier, which stage resonates most?
- Which is the highest stage you've experienced?
- Which is the lowest?
- Which stage (or stages) do you think you spend the most time in?

- What is your overall direction of travel? For instance, do you bounce between two earlier stages of burnout but not progress, or have you noticed you are gradually moving towards the later stages?
- Which stage do you currently identify with the most, and do you want to be there? If not, where do you want to be?

Resource 2: The Burnout Assessment Tool

The second means of assessing whether you have burnout is by completing the abbreviated Burnout Assessment Tool, which I'm providing here. This is a 12-question quiz that will give you a score so you can categorise your current situation into one of three categories: not suffering from burnout, at risk of burnout, or suffering severe burnout. I invite you to work through the quiz now.

For each question, score yourself as follows:

1 – Never; 2 – Rarely; 3 – Sometimes; 4 – Often; 5 – Always.

1. At work, I feel mentally exhausted.
2. At the end of the work day, I find it hard to recover my energy.
3. At work, I feel physically exhausted.
4. I struggle to find any enthusiasm for work.
5. I feel a strong aversion to my job.
6. I'm cynical about what my work means to others.
7. At work, I have trouble staying focused.
8. When working, I have trouble concentrating.
9. I make mistakes at work because my mind is on other things.
10. At work, I feel unable to control my emotions.
11. I do not recognise myself in the way I react emotionally at work.
12. At work, I may overreact unintentionally.

When you have worked through the questions, add up your total score and then divide by 12 to find your average score (stick to two decimal points).

Finally, use the key below to establish whether your score identifies you as not suffering from burnout, at risk of burnout or having severe burnout.

Key for scores:

1–2.53 = Green – not suffering from burnout.
2.54–2.95 = Orange – at risk of burnout.
2.96–5 = Red – suffering severe burnout.

Assessing your results from Resources 1 and 2

Now you have your answers from Resources 1 and 2, let's take a look at what these results actually mean and some next step suggestions for you.

If you identify with Stage 1 or 2 in Resource 1 and/or your score is Green in Resource 2

Congratulations! You are not currently burned out, but you might be at risk of it if you work in a high-stress job. Monitor your stress levels and if you feel that things are starting to change for the worse, come back to these resources to reassess yourself.

You can use this book to do the vitally important work on prevention, too, by first assessing your workplace/individual risk factors (as outlined in Part I) and then coming up with a plan to help mitigate their effects on you. This work is fundamental to stop your slide into burnout.

I would also suggest that you still read and engage with Part III of this book (which is all about recovery), because so much of the advice for burnout recovery is just as relevant and helpful for burnout prevention too. While I have labelled Part III as recovery advice, there are still so many gems in there for those of you who are actively looking to manage your stress a bit better! If you'd like some more help navigating Part III, the following might be particularly helpful as starting points:

- **Phase One, pp. 118–40:** The therapy-based techniques here are helpful for anyone who experiences stress and is looking for effective strategies to manage difficult or unwanted thoughts.

- **Step 4, pp. 141–47:** This section takes you through exercises to help work out your values, and how to engage with values-based decision-making. Everyone should read this section – burned out or not – because going through this process will help you to make vital, effective decisions about your work and career direction.
- **Step 5, pp. 147–69:** This section is about exploring career options. It is perfect for anyone that is looking to make changes to their career to prevent burnout or simply to work out the next career steps for you. (Don't miss out the section on writing a career development plan!)
- **Step 6, pp. 171–91:** This section takes you through how you can make an effective decision about your future career, how to successfully implement changes and maintain these changes to prevent burnout.
- **Two bonus steps** are provided to help you stay healthier after change and to identify and overcome barriers to change.

If you identify with Stage 3 in Resource 1 and/or your score is Orange in Resource 2

This is a position where you haven't burned out yet, but you're on your way. If this is you, then you have a wonderful opportunity to stop, take stock and make changes that will help to prevent things from getting worse. Everything discussed in Part III of this book will help you with this, so I encourage you to read on! You're in the right place.

What to do if you identify with Stages 4 or 5 in Resource 1 and/or your score is Red in Resource 2

If this is you, then you have severe burnout. Please consider getting urgent help from your doctor or therapist. Your immediate priority is getting expert help, taking time off from work (if available to you) and physically resting. I would strongly recommend that you do this before continuing to read this book. Your energy levels for engaging with reading will be low at this point of burnout, and you need to use what precious capacity you have to prioritise your recovery.

External help isn't always immediately or easily accessible, in which case (provided you do not have any symptoms of a mental health crisis, *see* p. 15 for a list of symptoms), I would suggest you start reading Steps 1–3 of your burnout recovery plan (which begins on p. 118) and take the advice from there.

Chapter 4 Takeaways

- The five stages of burnout include: the honeymoon phase, onset of stress, chronic stress, burnout and habitual burnout.
- The Burnout Assessment Tool is an excellent way of assessing and quantifying where you are at present: not suffering from burnout, at risk of burnout or suffering severe burnout.
- From these two resources you can work out whether you need help and what your next steps should be.

Is someone in your life burned out?

So far, we've only talked about how to recognise burnout in yourself, but I imagine there are some of you reading this now who are concerned about someone else in your life. This is the chapter for you.

Supporting Others with Burnout

The kicker in burnout is that often the person experiencing it doesn't realise how bad things are until they get to Stage 4 or 5 on the 'five stages of burnout' (as outlined on p. 96). Even though the signs and symptoms of the slide into burnout are significant, often the person that is in the thick of it might not realise what is happening until it's too late. Loved ones, close friends and colleagues will therefore often notice the changes before the burned-out person does.

Former tech co-founder and Head of Engineering, Dan Bartlett explains:

Burnout creeps up on you. If you were dropped straight into the boiling water of burnout, you'd immediately recoil. But when it heats up over time, it's really difficult to see what's happening.

Spotting Signs of Burnout in Others

From the outside, burnout in others might look like:

- **Social withdrawal:** Not spending as much time with friends and family, missing meetings at work, not engaging in small talk with colleagues.
- **Reduced performance at work:** Missing deadlines, taking longer to do things, working longer hours.
- **Behavioural changes:** Being snappy, irritable, grumpy or any other persistent negative change from their normal/baseline behaviour.
- **Unhealthy coping mechanisms:** You might notice the signs of increased alcohol consumption or substance misuse.

Talking to a Burned-out Person

If you would like to help a burned-out person, this will most likely begin with having a conversation with them. This has the potential to be a difficult conversation because the denial will be real. Raising concerns about burnout with someone who is developing it has to be approached with sensitivity and care.

Ask yourself: are you the right person to have this conversation? If this person is a work colleague, it might be that their supervisor or another trusted senior might be better. If you are a friend, would it be helpful to discuss things with the burned-out person's partner? If you are their partner, it might be that you are the best person for the job, however daunting that might feel.

I recommend having a gentle, non-judgemental conversation with the burned-out person to start. Pick a time and a place where neither of you are stressed or have other things to be doing. Privacy will be important, as the burned-out person might not feel safe to open up if there are lots of others around.

Start simply by asking how they are doing. Almost inevitably, they will tell you that things are fine. Alternatively, they might say that things aren't great, but they'll likely brush it off or minimise how they're feeling. If this happens, ask them how they are *really* doing. You could say that you've noticed their behaviour has changed, and that you're worried about them.

If they open up to you, try not to put your own perspective on to what they're experiencing. Simply listen and validate what they are telling you. There will likely be tears because often the burned-out person will have been feeling awful for some time. I would listen, recognise and validate their feelings, and then share resources and services to help them to get help.

If they deny any problems or decline help, leave them with the reassurance that you'll be there for them if things get worse. Signposting to available services might also be helpful, so when they realise what's happening to them, they know where to go for help.

Before you have this conversation, it would be good for you to know what services are available and how to access them. If you are having a conversation with someone that you work with, reminding them of what workplace well-being offerings are available will be helpful. If they are a loved one, and you're not sure what services are available at their work, remind them that they can talk to their doctor, or suggest speaking to their occupational health department. You could even suggest buying this book, or give a copy to them. If you are a friend or a colleague, then offering the burned-out person opportunities to socialise without any pressure or expectation to open up is also helpful.

How Can You Support Yourself?

If and when you decide to help a burned-out person, please remember that your own mental well-being is important, too! It might be difficult for you to shoulder the burden of the burned-out person's suffering alone, so make sure that you are signposting them to get help from the experts. You do not need to be their sole support.

In addition, knowing what you are available for (from an emotional perspective), and what you do not have capacity for is helpful, as this will help you to set effective boundaries as to how and when you are available for the burned-out person. If you'd like to know more about how to create empathetic boundaries, please skip to p. 182.

You can be there for others, but if someone is unwilling to acknowledge the problem or to get help then there's not much more you can do other than offer support. Don't burden yourself with guilt if they're not able to make changes or accept their situation. Please know that the person you're helping will be grateful for your love and support, even if they're not capable of showing it to you right now. They're still in there, and they can recover.

Finally, don't be scared to reach out for help yourself if you find that you are getting stressed or burned out yourself.

Chapter 5 Takeaways

- Burnout is more obvious to friends and family before it is to the burned-out person.
- Signs of burnout in others include: social withdrawal, reduced performance at work, behavioural change and unhealthy coping mechanisms.
- Offer support by talking to the burned-out person with sensitivity and care. Make sure you are best placed to have the conversation and start by asking how they are doing. Clue yourself up on the support and services available to them and how to access them.
- Look after yourself and reach out for help if you find that you are getting stressed or burned out.

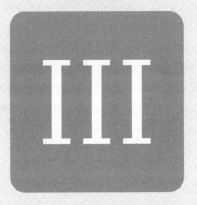

RECOVERY FROM BURNOUT: YOUR SIX-STEP RECOVERY PLAN

In this part of the book, I will be introducing you to my recommended six-step recovery plan. This is essential reading for anyone that identifies with being burned out, regardless of where you are in terms of your recovery. (It also contains great advice for those at risk of burnout with ways to effectively prevent burnout from happening; *see* pp. 102–3 for my advice on sections that may be particularly helpful if this is you.)

If you have only just realised that you're burned out, I recommend you begin with Step 1. I know that you will likely be struggling with fatigue and having difficulty with concentrating and motivation in the early days, so feel free to dip in and out as your energy level allows.

For everyone else – if you are already a few weeks or months into your recovery journey – I recommend you read through the overview of the six steps of burnout recovery (below), so you can work out where you currently are. This will help to inform your next steps and what you should be prioritising to help you progress. Everything that you learn here will complement any medical or psychological support you have, or it will give you some starting points if you can't currently access external care.

About the Six-Step Recovery Plan

Research on burnout has identified six common steps of burnout recovery. However, from my own work as a burnout specialist, I have found discussing these six steps within the context of three distinct recovery phases is helpful too, so that's what I'll do here. Burnout recovery is not linear, and it's perfectly normal to bounce back and forth between the six steps on your way to recovery. Adding in the three phases helps to give people the space they need to move through their recovery steps without feeling demoralised if they find themselves going 'backwards' at any point.

I have also found, from my own recovery journey, that there is some extra work that is helpful to do to help us stay healthy after recovery and supports us in identifying and overcoming any barriers to change. I include this as 'bonus' work with my patients. I'll include this bonus content here for you after the six steps, although you can visit this information at any time that feels right for you.

Let me give you an overview now of the six steps and then we'll dive into the detail.

> ### YOUR SIX-STEP RECOVERY PLAN: AN OVERVIEW
>
> **PHASE ONE: Getting healthy**
> - **Step 1**: Admitting there is a problem (*see* p. 118)
> - **Step 2**: Distancing from work (*see* p. 122)
> - **Step 3**: Restoring your health (*see* p. 125)
>
> **PHASE TWO: Preparing for change**
> - **Step 4**: Questioning your values (*see* p. 141)
> - **Step 5**: Exploring work possibilities (*see* p. 147)
>
> **PHASE THREE: Actioning change**
> - **Step 6**: Making changes at work (*see* p. 171)
> - **Bonus Step 1**: Staying healthy after change (*see* p. 192)
> - **Bonus Step 2**: Identifying and overcoming barriers to change (*see* p. 205)

The Six-Step Recovery Plan in More Detail

Now let's take a closer look at each step in more detail.

Phase One: Getting Healthy

This first phase of recovery is about acknowledging your problem and restoring your physical and mental health. Burnout takes a huge toll on your body, so here you stop, take stock and rest. You need to build up your energy again before you can do anything else, so this is what the work within this phase is focused on. Get this phase right and you'll set yourself up well for the rest of your post-burnout life and career. Phase One consists of Steps 1 to 3.

Step 1: Admitting There is a Problem

It is surprisingly hard to recognise burnout in yourself, but (like many other problems) the first step is acknowledging that you have a problem. At this point, it's usually very obvious to friends and family that you are in trouble, but you need to admit the situation to yourself and understand that things have to change.

As Kirsty Sinclair explains:

> *I was probably the last person to realise how unwell I was at the time. I was frightened to see it. I didn't know anyone else who had experienced burnout, as it wasn't the topic of conversation that it is now. It wasn't until I read advice in an online forum that suggested I open the curtains every day, I realised that someone else understood, had been through a similar state and had managed to survive it.*

Step 2: Distancing from Work

At this stage – in an ideal world – having a psychological and physical break from work is what we would be aiming for. For people who manage to achieve this, it's mainly through taking sick leave (sometimes for as long as a year, but on average it's for three and a half months), while others achieve a break by leaving their job entirely.

I do know that not everyone has the luxury of being able to take paid sick leave or leave their jobs, so don't panic if this is not for you! While it's not ideal from a recovery perspective, the good news is that many people do continue to work throughout their burnout recovery, so it is possible to feel better while continuing to work. (It might be reassuring to know that I did not stop working as a doctor during both my first and second burnout – and I still recovered!)

Step 3: Restoring Your Health

After acknowledging you have a problem and distancing yourself from work (if possible), it's time to focus on health. Fatigue is a significant burnout symptom, so this stage of recovery is about respecting that fatigue deficit. Most people at this stage sleep excessively, either by sleeping longer overnight or by taking frequent naps.

Besides sleep, people also engage in low-energy activities, such as watching TV or playing mindless games on their phones. After the initial fatigue starts to improve, people can gradually start to engage in fun activities, such as their hobbies, seeing friends and family socially, and physical activities. The goal at this stage is to restore energy levels and improve your mental and physical health.

Phase Two: Preparing for Change

After Phase One, you'll now have the energy in Phase Two to prepare to make changes to how you work. This involves doing some deep work on your new post-burnout values, and exploring every change you could make that would prevent burnout happening again.

How you approach this phase will very much depend on your personal circumstances:

- **If you're on sick leave**, you will simply be thinking about these changes.
- **If you're about to return to work**, you will need to think about what changes you need to make prior to your return.
- **If you are still working**, you will need to think about the changes you need while simultaneously balancing your workload.

Phase Two consists of Steps 4 and 5.

Step 4: Questioning Your Values

At this point, having regained some energy from Phase One, people reflect on their old values (and why they previously found them important) and then replace them with new values to support their recovery.

Your values act as your internal moral and ethical compass. Burnout is a lot like other significant life events, such as getting married, having a baby, a big bereavement or a divorce, in that it will cause you to question what is really important to you.

One common change during this particular stage is that everyone ultimately ends up placing more emphasis on their health. This stage of questioning your values is really important because every subsequent decision that you make needs to be based on what is now important to you post-burnout.

Step 5: Exploring Work Possibilities

Here, people work hard to research job opportunities that align with their new post-burnout values. This could be exploring the idea of continuing in your pre-burnout role with changes to suit your new values or it could mean looking for something completely new. This stage is about exploring rather than doing, though. It's about looking at every option that is open to you without the fear or burden of having to commit to anything just yet.

Phase Three: Actioning Change

While Phase Two is about researching and identifying the changes you need to make, Phase Three is all about action! This is about enacting the changes you need, then regularly reviewing them to ensure you stay well. Recovery is never straightforward and this phase is hard work, but it'll definitely be worth it to protect your hard-fought-for recovery.

I have included two bonus steps here that are not part of the official guidelines for recovering from burnout; instead this is extra information and techniques that I discovered on my own recovery journey and as a burnout specialist. I share this bonus content with my clients, so I want to share it with you too.

Step 6: Making Changes at Work

This step is about making changes to support your recovery – possibly the trickiest stage to get right and stay well during. This might mean changes to your existing job, leaving your job to step into a similar role in a different organisation, or even taking on something completely different in a new industry.

Some people need to leave the jobs that burned them out, but others don't. Your decision will very much depend on the reasons why you burned out, the changes that you've made to yourself, what's important to you now and what changes can be realistically made at work. For those that stay in their pre-burnout roles, implementing your professional boundaries is crucial for actioning successful change and, as such, we will cover this in depth.

In this section we'll go through how you can make an effective decision about your future career, how to successfully implement changes and how you can maintain these changes to secure your ongoing recovery.

Bonus Step 1: Staying Healthy After Change

Step 6 of burnout recovery is not the end of the recovery process but rather the start of a long journey back to full health after enacting changes at work. Maintaining your health after change requires ongoing effort and regular reviews – hence why I have added this section to the book. Here we will cover how to maintain your recovery after burnout through managing your stress levels and utilising your rest time and hobbies effectively.

Bonus Step 2: Identifying and Overcoming Barriers to Change

Early identification of any barriers to change will allow you to be far more effective and successful with any change you make. If you are looking to prevent burnout, then identifying and overcoming any barriers to change is helpful for guiding you through managing your stress.

While this section has been added as a bonus after the six steps, the advice given here can be used at any point:

- **If you have burnout**, this section can be used during any part of your recovery process, once you have completed Phase One.
- **If you chose to read this section during Phase Two**, anticipating any barriers in advance, before you implement change, will help you to mitigate them and improve your chances of a successful recovery.

- **If you chose to read this section during Phase Three**, the advice given here will help you to quickly spot and change any barriers that might prevent the changes you've put in place.

Before you Begin

Before you get started on your six-step recovery plan, I want to take a moment to acknowledge just how hard it is to go through recovery. At times, it will feel frustratingly slow, like you are taking one step forward and two steps back. But, trust me, you can and will get there.

I was completely clueless about everything I'm sharing in this section when I went through my own recovery process, so by empowering yourself with the knowledge of exactly what you need to do to get better, you're already way ahead. It's a hard process and you can normally expect each phase to last weeks or months at a time (with an overall recovery time of one to three years), but you can and will recover. I know this because I have recovered myself, and because I have supported many patients and clients to do so too.

I'll be sharing what to do at every step of burnout recovery, and I'll also be sharing where I went wrong at every stage. I'm being as open as I can be about this because I want things to be easier for you than they were for me.

Burnout recovery is not necessarily linear, and you are likely to bounce back and forth between steps at time. This is *totally normal* and to be expected. Please don't get disheartened if this happens to you, because it's all part of the process. Also, there's no hiding from the fact that burnout recovery is long, complex and needs to be multifaceted (i.e. you must make changes in multiple areas of your life and work for it to be successful and sustained). Therefore, it might look daunting when you're in the thick of it, but I'm here to guide you through every step of the way!

Exercise 28

 Identify your own needs

Read through the six steps of burnout recovery, and identify where you currently sit.

It's important to be able to identify this so that you know exactly what you need to be doing in this present moment to help yourself. You are welcome to skip to the relevant section for you if you prefer, but I would highly recommend that you read through *all* the steps from start to finish to ensure that you haven't missed anything that is going to be crucial to your recovery!

PHASE ONE: GETTING HEALTHY

Step 1: Admitting There is a Problem

My advice about what to do when you realise you are experiencing burnout is simple:

1. **Stop.**
2. **Take sick leave** (if this is available to you). If you cannot do this, have a conversation with your work about some immediate reasonable adjustments to help ease the load. You could also consider taking some annual leave, but please note that one or two weeks off work is not likely to be sufficient enough to kick-start recovery.
3. **Seek expert help**, either from a doctor or a therapist. If this is not an option, please don't worry, I have notes for you about this in the following pages. Reminder: if you are experiencing any suicidal tendencies or thoughts of self-harm, please seek same-day or urgent care.
4. **Give yourself a metaphorical, tearful, compassionate hug.** Well done. The first step of acknowledging there is a problem is *so* hard, but you're doing it.

This first step is simply about admitting you have a problem. At this point, you are not likely to have the energy or motivation to do much for yourself or others. Let go of any expectations you may have and be kind to yourself.

If you have loved ones around you then allow them to wrap you up in the warmth of their care. Let them take over tasks such as cooking and cleaning to help ease the burden on you, so you can concentrate on doing the things that really matter right now, i.e. physically resting.

If you don't have people around, I would suggest keeping your life as simple as possible and easing the load in other ways. This might mean outsourcing tasks such as the cleaning (if you have the financial means), ordering a takeaway, getting meal boxes delivered or buying ready-made meals so you don't need to cook for yourself. If you're a parent, it might mean finding extra childcare so that you can actually have some time to yourself (if this is available to you). It's all about reducing the everyday physical, mental and self-care load, as much as you can within your means, so that you can rest.

Kirsty Sinclair reflects on her own experience at this stage:

I was at home, knowing that my doctor and union were supporting my absence from work. I delegated what I could. I blocked all numbers linked to colleagues. Workplace access to me was filtered through my union rep, which helped reduce the cortisol levels. I had a small number of trusted people who contacted me regularly, and who were never offended if I didn't feel able to talk.

Remember, try not to beat yourself up about not recognising your burnout sooner. It's not your fault, you're not alone and you *will* get better.

Accessing Therapy

My standard advice would be that everyone with burnout should *ideally* have a course of tailored therapy, but I acknowledge that this is not an option for all. Not everyone has access to therapy and the wait times can be long, even for those who can access this support.

Please be assured that it is still possible to recover from burnout regardless of whether you have access to therapy or not. Therapy alone is not enough to recover from burnout, so while access to therapy is ideal, it is not the determining factor for a successful recovery.

A NOTE ON THERAPY AND USING THIS BOOK

This part of the book has been written to be helpful, regardless of whether you are able to access a therapist or not.

To summarise:

- **If you are able to see a therapist:** Great! The advice here is a fantastic add-on to the work you'll already be doing. I will take you through all the additional things you need to do outside of therapy to recover, and share the things I found particularly helpful during my own recovery.
- **If you are waiting to see a therapist:** The advice here will give you some simple therapy-based exercises and techniques to get started on while you wait. You can then continue using this as extra support to aid your ongoing recovery.
- **If you are unable to see a therapist:** This book will give you some simply therapy-based exercises and techniques to work with as you can. The advice here is not intended to replace seeing a therapist, but if you have barriers to access this support, it can certainly help.

What to Expect When Reaching out for Medical Support

It's pretty scary to ask for medical or psychological help in burnout, but there really is nothing to be afraid of. Here's an idea of what to expect from your doctor when you turn to them in a crisis.

Your doctor will normally begin by asking you questions about the pressures you're under right now, how this has made you feel and how it's been affecting your function and outlook. You can expect lots of questions therefore about your mood, feelings, sleep, eating patterns and whether you're drinking alcohol or using recreational drugs to cope.

Your doctor will also want to know what your home life is like: any responsibilities you may have at home and if you have anyone who is able to support you during this difficult time.

Expect to be asked if you have had any thoughts of suicide or self-harm, because it's your doctor's professional obligation to ensure your safety. If you do have any thoughts of suicide or harming yourself, your doctor will want to know who or what is keeping you safe and they will likely ask you some more detailed questions to get an idea of your level of risk. They will then decide if you need to have urgent mental health support, or whether you are safe to be managed 'in the community' (medical speak for 'at home', or for those that are outpatients using standard services such as seeing a therapist). If you are safe to be managed 'in the community', your doctor may offer advice about how to manage your symptoms (this might include changes to your lifestyle or a referral to appropriate services, such as talking therapies), sick notes for work and medication if appropriate.

How you answer all these initial questions will determine the next steps. Don't worry about crying in front of your doctor – this happens more often than you might think and doctors are always there to support.

What to Expect from Therapy

The type and structure of therapy you may be offered is likely to depend on what's available in your local area. Typically, for burnout, you might expect 10 hour-long sessions delivered virtually or in person (although depending on your symptoms you might be offered more or less). Both CBT (*see* p. 133) and ACT (*see* p. 136) are helpful in burnout. As Dan Bartlett reflects:

> *Despite my scepticism, a few sessions of CBT had a big impact. While the intense demands of work had been the primary factor in my burnout, CBT helped me see how my thinking was still perpetuating a feeling of exhaustion and exasperation through repeating variants of the storyline that 'Everything is terrible, I don't have the energy, what's the point?'*

Your therapist will assess your symptoms and how much they are affecting you. You might be asked to do a questionnaire to help with this.

(Normally, at least the first session will be dedicated to completing this questionnaire.) Then you will start the therapy.

During the sessions, your therapist will talk you through exercises they believe will help you, and then it will be up to you to practise them outside of the sessions. I have included a few of my favourite therapy exercises to help in burnout on p. 129.

Therapy sessions are likely to feel intense and draining in the moment, but I suggest you view the exercises given to you in therapy as though it is physio for the mind: the exercises are most powerful when done regularly and consistently outside of the therapy room.

Step 2: Distancing From Work

Steps 1 and 2 often happen concurrently or in rapid succession. In Step 2, it's important to distance yourself from the work – both physically and metaphorically – that led you to burnout.

Options for this might include:

* taking sick leave;
* taking annual leave (while this is not likely to be sufficient to recover from burnout, it would give you a temporary break from your work stress);
* leaving your current role (either for a new role within your company or moving elsewhere);
* taking a break from work altogether.

Whatever your situation, the key is to distance yourself from the source of the stress (i.e. your current work) in whatever way is possible for you, so that you can start the recovery process. You should expect this stage to last some weeks, if not months, as even if you are able to remove yourself physically from work fairly quickly (i.e. taking sick leave), it can take time to remove yourself mentally.

Ideally, during burnout recovery, removing yourself from any form of work completely is the best option, but in the modern day this is difficult to achieve. Financially, most people now have to work, so leaving the workforce altogether is very rarely an option.

Even if you can access sick leave, you will likely need to have some contact with your work to keep the lines of communication open about your progress and your return (although it's important that you are not contacted too regularly or are made to feel that you are being hounded, especially in the early days).

The study that originally outlined the six steps of burnout recovery was conducted back in 1998 (although the work still stands). However, the communication landscape was very different back then, so when people went on sick leave in the 1990s there was no access to work emails, mobile phones, WhatsApp or Slack. So, I encourage you to turn off your email and notifications, and retreat to somewhere safe, physically and metaphorically.

I can't afford to take sick leave or leave my job... what should I do?

I get asked this question a lot. As outlined above, I think it's important to flag that the 'ideal' circumstance for burnout recovery is to take time off work, but I know that's not possible for many of us. Not everyone has the financial security of paid sick leave, and taking unpaid time off work might not be an option, particularly during the current cost-of-living crisis. Finding a new job while you're already feeling burned out might also not be possible for you. So what does that mean?

It will hopefully be reassuring for you to hear that research conducted into burnout recovery over recent years suggests first that most people do have to continue to work throughout their burnout and recovery period, and second that a change of workplace or job has not been found to be a decisive factor when it comes to a successful recovery period. Burnout recovery is complex and there is no single act (like leaving the job that's causing the burnout) that will fix it. Leaving your current workplace that causes you stress is therefore ideal for your burnout recovery but it's not essential, so don't panic.

Personally, I didn't take any sick leave with my first period of burnout and recovery, and I continued to work in the role that had caused my burnout until I left it six months after my first panic attack. This was down to the difficult combination of my work asking me not to go off sick, coupled with the internalised pressure that I put on myself to keep working. It was only when I started to slide back into burnout for the second time that I was forced to take myself out of full-time NHS (public sector) work for nine months to allow for adequate recovery. However, I continued to work part-time as a private GP during this period, as the working environment was completely different. As such, I found the pressures manageable.

Everyone's experience of burnout is unique. If sick leave or a job change is available to you, please take it and don't allow yourself to be consumed with guilt over it (more on guilt to come, *see* p. 214).

If removing yourself from the current role that is burning you out is not an option, there are three factors you can concentrate on instead. Mastering these are the three key predictors of a successful burnout recovery, and they're probably not what you might think (you may remember having discussed them earlier in Part I). They are:

1. Having control/agency at work (*see* 'Control', p. 41)
2. Believing that you are in control of your well-being (*see* 'Control', p. 41)
3. Good relationships (*see* 'Community', p. 49)

That's it. If you focus on *nothing* else but work on improving these three factors alone, you are more likely to have a successful burnout recovery, even if you do need to remain in your current role.

The reason why these three factors are so powerful is because if you believe that you have control at work and over your well-being, you're much more likely to bring about the changes needed to ensure you recover (Exercise 4 can help with control, *see* p. 42). Then having good, supportive relationships – or at least one safe, solid relationship with a partner, family member or friend – will help you with accountability and provide a safe space to offload.

So, if you are unable to successfully distance yourself from the work that is burning you out, don't lose hope. Ideally, yes, a period of sick leave is helpful, but if this is not available to you then you have options. You can still make changes that will positively impact on your recovery. It might take a little longer and need a bit more work from you to get there, but it's definitely achievable.

Step 3: Restoring Your Health

This next step is all about restoring your mental and physical health. This is essential to master because you need to rebuild your energy before you can move forward any further.

Restoring your mental and physical health might take weeks or months to achieve – it cannot be rushed. If you follow my advice on how to loosely structure this step, you will increase your chances of successfully restoring your health as quickly as possible, while also reducing the risk of slipping back into ill health through burnout again.

Why Is Rest So Important?

In this third step of burnout recovery, your restoration of health begins with rest. Rest is crucial in this early stage because people begin their burnout recovery with very low energy.

The Effort-Recovery Theory

To help get your head around the importance of rest at this stage, let's talk about a helpful concept called the effort-recovery theory, which explains how burnout can be accelerated and made worse by daily activities.

Your work-related activities require cognitive and physical energy to complete – in other words, there's a cost. Imagine you have a pot of money and are going to work and spending that money on doing your work tasks. This cost can be recovered after a brief break from work, so when you rest, you get more money back in your energy pot. If the break is too short, or never taken, the cost is never recovered. In the run-up to burnout, imagine you are spending your energy money and it's not being replenished.

When an employee with an energy deficit approaches work-related tasks, their productivity will be reduced and they will work more slowly. To make up for the shortfall, the employee might work overtime, which again prevents recuperation from the cost of work-related activities. As a result, the employee is continuously working at an energy loss and can never fully recuperate, which can ultimately lead to burnout.

I think this effort-recovery concept helps to explain *why* adequate rest is really important in burnout recovery, as people who are burned out will have *huge* energy deficits and considerable, disproportionate fatigue. It's therefore important that you use any time you can to rest so you can recoup some of those costs, which will help with your recovery.

The effort-recovery theory tells us that people recover from burnout when their cognitive and physical resources are recharged; in other words, when they've received enough rest. I know so many of us who are burned out can identify with the feeling of energy depletion, both mentally and emotionally. Therefore, rest is absolutely key in your burnout recovery.

The Recovery Paradox

Let me share with you now a second theory that helps to demonstrate the importance of rest at this stage. Research shows that the more we're struggling with our health, the less likely we are to engage in activities to help ourselves. This is what's known as the 'recovery paradox'.

In burnout, when work is demanding and overwhelming, it is very easy to revert to a negative cycle of working more and taking fewer breaks. That's certainly what I did when I burned out. In addition, when going through a stressful time you are less likely to eat nutritiously or drink enough water. You might even turn to alcohol or other substances to help you cope. Essentially, because of your stress you are not in the right emotional place to successfully engage in good, healthy behaviours. Further depleted from these negative cycles, you are going to have even less energy and motivation to take time out to relax or engage in exercise and other healthy activities. This then leads to low chances of recovery and, in turn, further exhaustion. It becomes an exhausting self-perpetuating cycle, known as the recovery paradox.

This is what we typically see in burnout. People get themselves into a huge crisis and struggle with their symptoms. When you are in this position and need change the most, it's actually the time when you have the least capacity to make the changes you need. This is why rest is so key during the early stages of burnout. You have to be well-rested mentally and physically before you can begin to work your way further through the burnout recovery cycle and begin to tackle the root cause of your burnout.

There is quite literally no point in trying to attempt anything in the latter stages of the burnout recovery cycle when you are early on in your recovery. None whatsoever. Don't worry yourself stupid about what on earth you are going to do for the rest of your working life until you have gone through the process of resting, recovering and starting to engage in the things you enjoy (as outlined in Steps 1–3).

Activities to Help You Rest

In the early stages of recovery (i.e. Step 1 to early Step 3), it is crucial that downtime activities are *not* outcome driven. They should require little effort and should be purely enjoyable (it might be difficult to get enjoyment from any activity if you're really burned out – hang on in there, it does get better). Importantly, activities at this stage should allow for rest.

Activities to allow for rest include:

- sleeping more and napping;
- watching TV;
- playing instinctive and intuitive games (requiring little brainpower) on your phone or tablet;
- mindful colouring.

As you move through Step 3, you will slowly begin to feel a little better and more rested. At this point, the burnout literature suggests you focus on activities that allow for socialisation and get you moving.

Activities That Allow for Socialisation

Truthfully, when you're burned out, it's hard to motivate yourself to go back into social activities, especially when you're struggling to engage with basic self-care, such as showering or brushing your teeth. However, it is something that you should be prioritising because it *will* help.

The goal of social interactions with friends and family is to develop healthy support networks. We know that social connection and peer support are really important in burnout recovery. If you're anything like me, you will probably not want to see too much of other people at this stage, but the science is quite clear that it will help you to feel better.

You could start by seeing a small number of close and trusted people for short periods of time. If you're not up for talking about your burnout, simply make that clear before you see them so there are no crossed wires or awkward moments!

Activities to Get You Moving

Regularly taking part in exercise and sport can reduce the harmful effects of stress. Exercise also helps with healthy behaviour seeking, and will impact positively on other aspects of burnout, such as poor sleep. Researchers advise exercising in a group with friends when you can, because then you're simultaneously doing a social activity with a physical activity.

Start small and build up, if you're struggling with motivation. For instance, if a daily walk is accessible to you but you can't get the motivation to get out, start by putting your shoes by the front door. The next day, change into the shoes, open the door and stand in the doorway for five minutes. The following day, do the same, but challenge yourself to walk to the end of the road. You could enlist the help of a friend and go for a walk with them. This is just one example of how you can achieve some realistic exercise in burnout, but what you pick to do and how you go about it is entirely up to you. Just ensure the exercise is appropriate for your energy levels, accessible for your present lifestyle and one that you might even enjoy!

You don't need to do high-impact or high-intensity exercise to get the benefits (at this stage, high-intensity exercise wouldn't be that helpful as it doesn't respect your fatigue deficit). It's more important to be doing something that fits in with your lifestyle and gets you moving – anything is better than nothing! As you start to feel better, you can begin to engage in activities that are more physical and require more energy, but take it slow. You are likely to feel fatigued after exerting yourself at this stage, so ensure that the things you do are graded (starting small and short with long periods of rest between activities). Over time, you can gradually up the duration and length of the activities and shorten the periods of rest. How quickly you do this is unique to you and your symptoms, but what I can say is that regardless of how long it takes, you will want it to be faster and it will feel frustrating! Don't rush. Respect your symptoms and pull back if you overexert yourself.

At this stage of your recovery, you will have limited energy and resources so you would be right to ask yourself where to use those limited resources for maximum-recovery returns. Burnout gets better with low-energy, social and physical activities, *but* if you have high burnout scores or are early on in your recovery, the most beneficial way to recover, according to the data, is to engage in social activities followed by 'low-cost' activities. The important thing to remember is that the severity of your burnout will determine how well you respond to these measures and when you should do them.

Therapeutic Exercises to Support Phase One

Ideally, everyone in burnout recovery would be engaging with a psychologist and going through a course of therapy, but we know that's not accessible for many of us. Therefore, I'm sharing with you now a selection of five different exercises for you to choose from, all of which will help you start to feel better.

These exercises are a compilation of the CBT and ACT exercises that helped me the most during my own burnout recovery. Truthfully (and don't tell my therapist this!), I was initially sceptical about how much these exercises would help me. But I knew more than anything that I wanted to get better and I would have done pretty much anything at that point to make the burnout go away. I therefore threw myself into engaging with therapy, despite my reservations, and I ended up being blown away by the positive impact these exercises had.

When I completed my course of therapy, I was nervous about being able to stay well without the guidance of my therapist. However, I have continued to use the techniques I learned and I am pleased to report that they have kept me in good stead during my recovery. It's really taught me that you cannot approach therapy with a 'one and done' attitude – therapeutic practices are techniques that will help you for the rest of your life, and they need to be done regularly for you to stay well.

I'm providing you here with a selection of CBT- and ACT-based techniques to get you started with your burnout recovery. Read through all of them first, then pick one or two techniques to start practising regularly this week and see how you get on. Remember that you must do these regularly to notice any improvements, and it does take time (I'd recommend practising them whenever you experience a difficult thought or emotion). Give it a chance, but if you find that a particular technique is not helping, please try one of the other exercises or seek one-to-one therapy, if possible.

DISCLAIMER

Although I am trained in ACT, I am not a clinical psychologist and these exercises are not a replacement for a one-to-one course of therapy. Having a course of therapy means that what is discussed with you is tailored to your particular needs and circumstances, and having an interaction with a therapist can also hold you accountable.

I cannot offer you individual therapy here, but what I will be sharing now might be sufficient for some of you to get started, at least. It might even be sufficient to allow you to feel well enough to progress on to the next stage in your recovery.

As a reminder, I also do not recommend using this book (or any therapy book) if the way you're feeling right now is severely affecting your function, or if you feel you are at risk of harm or suicide. Please seek urgent face-to-face medical attention if this is the case.

Unhelpful Styles of Thinking

Discovering unhelpful thinking styles was one of the first techniques that I encountered in my own therapy journey, and it felt like a real revelation. I knew my thoughts were negative but I had no idea I was engaging with pretty much every unhelpful style of thinking possible (no wonder my head was such a horrifically exhausting place to exist).

The ten unhelpful styles of thinking are as follows:

1. **Black-and-white thinking:** 'If I'm not perfect then I have failed' – thinking in extremes.
2. **Overgeneralising:** 'Everything is rubbish', 'there's no point' – seeing a pattern based upon a single event or being overly broad in the conclusions drawn.
3. **Mental filter:** Only paying attention to certain types of evidence; for example, solely seeing your shortcomings or failures.
4. **Disqualifying the positive:** 'That doesn't count' – discounting the good things that have happened or that you have done.
5. **Jumping to conclusions:** Mind reading, i.e. assuming we know what other people are thinking, and fortune telling – predicting the future.
6. **Catastrophising and minimising:** Either blowing things out of proportion or inappropriately shrinking something to make it seem less important.

7. **Emotional reasoning:** 'I feel embarrassed, so I must be an idiot' – assuming that because we feel a certain way that it must be true.

8. **Critical thinking:** Using critical words such as 'should', 'must' or 'ought'.

9. **Labelling:** 'I'm a loser', 'They're such an idiot' – assigning labels to ourselves or others.

10. **Personalisation:** 'This is my fault' – blaming yourself or taking responsibility for something that isn't completely your fault or, blaming other people for something that was your fault.

Exercise 29

Identifying unhelpful styles of thinking

This exercise will help us to identify any unhelpful styles of thinking we may be engaging with, so we know where improvements can be targeted.

Read through the list of unhelpful thinking styles above and identify if any are affecting you right now. If so, which ones are affecting you the most?

Capturing Negative Associated Thoughts

Have you ever thought, 'I'm terrible at my job', 'I'm a failure', 'I'm a terrible person' or 'I'm letting everyone down'? Quite often these negative and anxious thoughts feed into burnout and then get worse with burnout, too. In burnout, difficult thoughts will have a significant impact on your mood and function, and they'll stop you from helping yourself.

These thoughts can be automatic and habitual, so they just pop into your mind (in other words, you don't decide to think of them, they just happen). They seem to be believable facts, so you tend to accept them at face value. However, they are actually highly biased. Even though these thoughts might seem right to you, they are likely to be distorted or inaccurate. They might support some of your feelings or things that have happened, but they ignore many other factors that do not fit in with that negative view. Therefore, in burnout, you can get tunnel vision where you can see nothing but these negative thoughts.

Learning to identify the negative thoughts that commonly show up for you will allow you to form arguments against them. This in turn will help you to change your patterns of thinking and will assist your recovery. Learning how to catch these negative thoughts can be quite difficult at first. These thoughts may have become such a habit that you do not recognise them as being negative.

To learn how to catch these thoughts, I recommend that you use your feelings as a cue. Whenever you notice that you're feeling upset or your mood takes a downturn, ask yourself, 'What was going through my mind just then?' Or if you don't 'hear' thoughts in your head, think, 'What did I see in my head?' instead. If you seem to be upset, angry or distressed by a situation, ask yourself: 'How did I view the situation?' and 'What did this mean to me?' Hopefully, by questioning yourself in this way, you can start to get an idea about what your negative thoughts were and what prompted them.

Now that you have an idea about which unhelpful styles of thinking you have been experiencing, let's look at ways to effectively reduce the impact of these unhelpful styles of thinking. To do this, I'll be taking you through two CBT-based and two ACT-based exercises.

WHAT IS CBT?

Cognitive Behavioural Therapy, or CBT, is a type of talking therapy that teaches you coping skills for dealing with different problems. It deals with how you think and behave, and helps you turn negative thoughts into more positive ones. I'm going to share the very first CBT technique I was taught by my own therapist now, because it was so helpful to me early on in my therapy journey.

Exercise 30

Capturing your negative associated thoughts (CBT)
When you are not feeling good, ask yourself these questions to help you identify your automatic, negative thoughts:

- What was going through my mind just before I started to feel this way?
- What does this say to me?
- If it were true, what does this mean about me, my life and my future?
- What am I afraid might happen?
- What's the worst thing that could happen if it were true?
- If it were true, what does this mean about the other person or people in general?

Keeping a Thought Diary

Once you have started to capture your negative thoughts from Exercise 30, the next step is to keep them in a diary and to write down the evidence that does and does not support each thought. The idea here is that we're challenging the automatic belief with evidence.

I kept a thought diary for a few weeks and every time I felt upset, sad, confused or distressed, I wrote down my negative thoughts and went through the process of writing down alternatives. With time, it became quicker and easier, to the point where I now no longer need to write everything down, but I do it internally. Like anything new, it takes time to practise and refine the skill. It's worth the effort, though, because this really will help to change how you think, feel and behave.

Write down your thought as it is, then write yourself an alternative, more balanced thought. Focus on this alternative thought, then ask yourself: 'How am I feeling now?' You can capture this information using a table, such as the one opposite (I have filled in an example for you):

Where were you/ describe the situation	Emotion or feeling	Negative thought	Evidence that supports the thought	Evidence that does not support the thought	Alternative thought	Emotion or feeling
I made a mistake at work.	Stressed and anxious.	I'm a failure. I'm incompetent at my job. They're going to fire me.	My boss has asked for a meeting to discuss the mistake. No one else on the team has made this mistake.	The last time I made a mistake I was well supported to learn from it and improve. The majority of my work is at a very high standard. My boss is supportive and no one else has been fired for making a mistake.	It is human to make mistakes and unreasonable to expect perfection in every bit of work that I do. I am going to use this as an opportunity to reflect, learn, make changes and improve my work.	Less stressed. Still concerned about the meeting, but feeling like I can go in having reflected, and feeling prepared.

Exercise 31

Keeping a thought diary (CBT)

Keep a thought diary for seven days, then assess how you now feel. Have you noticed any patterns or common themes that kept popping up? How did keeping the diary help you to form new thoughts and perspectives?

The idea with these CBT exercises is that – over time and with practice –it'll become much easier for you to identify your negative thoughts and come up with the evidence against them, so you can create alternative positive thoughts more quickly.

WHAT IS ACT?

Acceptance and Commitment Therapy (ACT) is different to CBT in that rather than challenging negative thoughts and forming alternative positive ones, as we do in CBT, ACT helps people to accept their unwanted thoughts but then commit to *action*.

In ACT, thoughts are not changed or even labelled as 'negative' or 'positive'; rather they are assessed as to whether they are helping you to achieve your goals and live the life you want.

The ultimate aim of ACT is to increase psychological flexibility, which simply means to be aware of any situation that you are in and the thoughts you are experiencing but then be able to take action, based not on unwanted thoughts but on your current goals and values.

Let's say that you are experiencing thoughts that you are really stressed and that you cannot cope with your current workload. You are overcome with these thoughts – so much so that you cannot start to make any changes at work in order to effectively deal with your workload. In ACT, you learn techniques to accept these thoughts.

Once you've done this, you would go and make changes to how you manage your workload in accordance with your goals and values (*see* p. 144 for more information on how to work out your values, and how to make effective decisions based on them). In this case, the goal might be that you want to stay at your place of work and find practical ways to ease the burden of your workload, and so your values-driven action could be that you arrange a meeting with your manager to discuss reasonable adjustments to help you manage your workload more effectively.

You can see here that ACT doesn't change your thoughts, rather it changes how you *react to* them. The idea is that you go on to make changes that should ultimately help you to live the life you want to live, in alignment with what is important to you.

Using Defusion to Manage Unwanted Emotions, Thoughts and Feelings

'Defusion' is an ACT-based technique that you can use whenever you're experiencing a difficult emotion, thought or feeling. I'm going to share my favourite defusion exercise with you here, using the sensation of feeling stressed as an example, but this can easily be adapted for any difficult feeling you are experiencing (for example guilt, anxiety or loneliness).

Exercise 32

 I'm having the thought that... (ACT)

1. Acknowledge the next time you feel really stressed by saying to yourself, 'I'm feeling stressed'. Sit with it. Repeat this in your head several times and see how you feel.

2. Change what you're saying in your head to, 'I'm having the thought that I am feeling stressed.' Repeat this in your head several times and observe how you feel.

3. Change what you're saying to yourself to, 'I'm observing that I am having the thought that I am feeling stressed.' Again, repeat this several times and see how you feel.

By doing this technique you can make space for the difficult emotion, thought or feeling that you are experiencing. Instead of getting 'hooked' by your negative thought (and letting it stop you from doing the things you want to be doing), you create a level of detachment between you and the thought so you can carry on achieving your goals.

This exercise does take a bit of practice, but it's incredibly powerful and helpful once you have mastered it. Remember, the aim is not to feel 'good' or 'better' but to simply make space for the thought, treat it without judgement and not to let it control your behaviour in a way that you don't want. With time and practice, you should be able to respond flexibly to uncomfortable thoughts and situations much more easily.

Other ways to practise defusion might include:

- **Thanking your mind:** Whatever your mind says – no matter how judgemental or horrible – warmly respond with, 'Thanks, mind!', and then redirect your energies into something more life-enhancing.
- **Naming the story:** Put your thoughts or feelings into a story. When you experience them, remind yourself, 'Oh, here's this story again.' For instance, you might label thoughts of self-doubt and low confidence as 'the I'm not good enough story'. You can even write it on a piece of paper and pull it out when you experience these feelings!
- **Sing your thought to yourself:** Use a silly voice or sing to the tune of 'Happy Birthday'.
- **Imagine the thought as a black type on a computer:** In your mind, play around with the colours and fonts.

Pick one or two of the above defusion exercises to try out this week and see if they work for you. Note that these challenges don't look to change the thought you're experiencing; instead, they allow you to respond flexibly to how you are thinking so that your thoughts can influence but not dominate your behaviours.

Grounding Your Emotions

If you are feeling overwhelmed with intense emotion of any kind (anything from sadness to anger), you might want to try a grounding technique like this 'dropping anchor' practice. The idea is not to change your intense emotions or thoughts, but instead to hold you steady until the emotional storm passes, in the same way that an anchor doesn't change stormy weather but steadies a boat until it passes.

The aim of the exercise below is *not* to feel better; it is to reflect on:

- whether you have more focus, control and presence;
- whether the thoughts are helpful or useful when tackling your problems or goals;
- what you need to do next in terms of values-based action, so that you can lead a rich and fulfilling life.

Exercise 33

Dropping anchor – a grounding technique (ACT)
The next time you feel overwhelmed with an intense emotion, try this exercise and see how you feel.

1. Sit in a chair and hold yourself still.
2. Close your eyes, acknowledge your thoughts and feelings then name and notice them. You could say to yourself, 'I am feeling anxious.'
3. Connect with your body and notice how it feels. Move a little and take control of your physical actions. You could take a stretch, push your feet gently into the floor or push your fingertips together.
4. Engage with the world by opening your eyes. Take a look around. What do you see? What do you hear? What can you feel?

How to know when Phase One is Complete

The amount of time that it will take for you to feel mentally and physically restored will be unique to you. Typically, Phase One lasts several weeks to months, so there's no need to rush it. There also isn't a defined moment when you should or will be ready to move to Phase Two.

Don't forget that Phase Two in your burnout recovery isn't about returning to work or beginning to action changes in the workplace (if you're still working). Rather, it focuses on *thinking* and *researching* possible changes at work, not actioning them. Therefore, you need energy to move to Phase Two but you don't need to be back to your previous state of function. You just need to be sufficiently recovered to engage in some thinking about your values and, following that, your work options.

It can be helpful to have a rough indicator of when you might want to think about the next steps. So, here are my suggestions for when you're ready to move forward to Phase Two:

- You start to feel that the mental fog is lifting and you are having more good days than bad.
- You're managing problems more effectively and are able to cope more easily.
- You're able to look after yourself rather than self-neglecting; for example, you can wash, cook and clean.
- You feel that you have a little bit of something left at the end of the day.
- You have mental and emotional capacity to effectively manage daily issues that arise.
- You do not get the 'fight or flight' response when thinking about work.
- You are starting to get the itch to work again – although please note that you will likely not feel motivated to go back to the job that burned you out. Instead, this will be more of a feeling that you are wanting the challenge, routine, purpose and interaction that work gives you.

PHASE TWO: PREPARING FOR CHANGE

Step 4: Questioning Your Values

One of the unintentional mistakes I made during my first burnout recovery was not understanding that there was a recovery process to follow, and as such I missed out some crucial stages. Step 4 and my revision of values was one of these because, being truthful, I just didn't know (at the time) that this was one of the key steps of successful burnout recovery.

As a result of inadvertently skipping Step 4, I denied myself permission to explore my new post-burnout values; instead, throughout my recovery and beyond, I was still driven by my old pre-burnout values. Every decision I made at the time was about duty and service and had me trying to stay in the full-time GP work that had aligned with these old values and burned me out. With time, I came to realise that duty and service were no longer my driving values, so those career choices were not going to work for me in the long run.

When I slid into burnout for a second time, I worked out what I'd missed in my recovery the first time round and made sure to prioritise those missing pieces. A big part of my second recovery was identifying my new values. Since then, every decision I have made has been in alignment with my new values, and I feel so much better. So, in summary, don't miss this step!

Why Values Matter

In Phase One, we covered how a mismatch between your personal values and the values of your employer is a key risk factor for the development of burnout – and if you don't feel valued by your employer this puts you at risk too (*see* p. 47). Therefore, after burnout occurs, it's important to revise your values in the same way that people do after other big life events, such as a bereavement, divorce, illness or becoming a parent.

Values are the principles that *you* personally deem to be a priority; by which you live your life and make decisions. They are your personal judgement of what is important in life and work, unique to you. Essentially, they are the things that you believe in and are important in determining your priorities. In this way, values help you to set effective goals and, deep down, they're probably the measures you use to tell if your life is turning out the way you want it to. Values provide direction for your decision-making and motivate you to make important changes.

When the things that you do and the way that you behave match your values, life is usually good – you're satisfied and content. But when your actions and decisions don't align with your personal values, that's when things can feel wrong. Not only can it feel wrong but, as we discussed in Part I (*see* p. 46), a mismatch of values can be a factor in burnout too. For instance, if you value family life but you have to work 70-hour weeks and always miss putting the kids to bed, you will inevitably feel internal stress and conflict. When I burned out, I valued spending time with my patients and I got a lot of satisfaction from feeling that I had the resources to do a good job, but I just couldn't do that under the conditions I was forced to work under. The subsequent moral injury of this was 100 per cent a factor in my burnout.

Values are usually fairly stable, yet they don't have strict limits or boundaries – for most of us, our values will evolve and change with time and life experiences. Studies have shown that burnout changes people's values too, and to me this makes complete sense. Burnout is a huge, cataclysmic event that significantly changes your emotional, mental and physical health, so it makes sense that it can alter your outlook on life. Interestingly, there is one common thing that happens to everyone that experiences burnout: they value their health more post-burnout.

The fact that our values evolve over time is why keeping in touch with them is a lifelong exercise – particularly so after burnout. Assessing your new values forms a crucial part of your burnout recovery but you should continuously revisit your values, especially if you start to feel unbalanced and you can't quite figure out why. In burnout, re-evaluating your values needs to happen in this step because Step 5 is when we begin to explore new work possibilities. You need to have your new values in place first to ensure any new work opportunities you consider align with these.

My Personal Values

Prior to my burnout, as I mentioned, I prioritised duty and service along with dependability, mastery and safety in my work. When my work started to put pressure on me and I felt I couldn't deliver on safe patient care, it caused huge internal pain because my values were being compromised. Post-burnout, my new values are: advocacy, family, autonomy, creativity and health. Let me share how I have incorporated these new values into my life:

- **Advocacy:** I do my advocacy work through my role as a charity ambassador for Doctors in Distress (https://doctors-in-distress.org .uk) and through sharing information about burnout and my own burnout journey on social media.
- **Family:** I've changed the way I work – and the hours I work – to be able to spend more time with my family, and to not have to stress about childcare and missed drop-offs and pick-ups.
- **Autonomy:** I cannot change the fundamental pressures at work that caused me to burn out, but I have been able to change the type of work I do and when I do it.
- **Creativity:** This has allowed me to explore mastery and getting into a state of flow, both of which are essential in burnout recovery (more about this in Bonus Step 1, *see* p. 196). I have achieved this through taking up sewing and embroidery, which I try to do once the kids are in bed. This avoids me getting sucked into watching too much Netflix!
- **Health:** I do, of course, value my health too. In every decision I make about my career now I ask myself, does this decision allow me to work in a way that will sustain my recovery?

Living my life in accordance with my new, changed values has helped me to create a work pattern that works for me and my family post-burnout. I realise that I am lucky in many respects because my job gives me a huge degree of flexibility, but being able to make these changes has been crucial to recovery.

Therapeutic Exercises to Reassess Your Values

The good news is that reassessing your values shouldn't take you too long. If you don't know how to go about this process, don't worry because I'm going to take you through exactly how to do this in the simplest way possible now. (I once did an online values quiz that took me through so many steps that after about 10 minutes, I gave up. I was still clueless about my values, and rather frustrated that it wasn't an easy process, to boot. But it really doesn't have to be that onerous.)

The important thing is that you are sufficiently recovered from Phase One and have restored your health enough to be able to engage in the process. Please don't try to do this stage too early in your recovery. So, when you're ready, let's get started.

How to Identify Your Own Personal Values

Opposite is a list of values. Your task is to simply look at the list and pick out the five values that are most important to you right now.

If you're like me, you'll find it hard to pick just five values because all of these are great! If this is you, I suggest picking ten values and then narrowing them down to five. Think about the times when you are most happy and fulfilled. At these times, which values stand out as the most important?

There is no judgement about which values matter most. For example, if you pick wealth over respect, it doesn't matter and it's no reflection on you and your worth as a person. What matters is that you are true to yourself. Also, you don't have to share your values with anyone (unless you want to), so the only person you need to be honest with is yourself.

Make your selection from the values listed now. If you don't find any – or enough – values that resonate, there are plenty of lists of values available online. Don't overthink this process – go with your gut instinct and spend a maximum of 15 minutes on this task.

- Accountability
- Achievement
- Adventure
- Altruism
- Authenticity
- Autonomy
- Balance
- Beauty
- Boldness
- Challenge
- Community
- Compassion
- Competence
- Contribution
- Creativity
- Curiosity
- Determination
- Fairness
- Faith
- Family
- Financial security
- Friendship
- Fun
- Generosity
- Growth
- Health
- Honesty
- Humour
- Inner Harmony
- Justice
- Kindness

- Knowledge
- Leadership
- Love
- Loyalty
- Openness
- Peace
- Resilience
- Respect
- Security
- Self-Care
- Service
- Spirituality
- Stability
- Status
- Success
- Trustworthiness
- Wealth
- Wisdom

Now you have selected your values, write them down so that you can refer to them when needed. The Notes app on your phone or a journal would work well for this, or you might prefer to have them somewhere more visible, such as on a note stuck on to your laptop. Wherever you choose to write down your values, keep this list safe because we'll need it again in Phase Three, when we look at making decisions about your post-burnout career direction.

How to Assess Your Company's Values

The next thing to think about is the values of the organisation you work for. At the time of writing this, I was sat in a branch of Costa (our home internet had gone down and I needed their Wi-Fi to work). So, let's look at their company values as an example. According to their website, the values of Costa are: passion, warmth, courage and trust. As I was researching internet providers, I noted that the values of Virgin Media are: brave, real and together, and one of the values of British Telecom is to 'fearlessly push for the highest standards'. Your company will also have values that should (in theory at least) permeate through the organisation and be clear at every level of the company.

Exercise 34

 Your values vs your company's values

1. Identify what your current company's values are. (These can usually be found on your company website.)
2. Consider if your company actually lives by its intended values?
3. Compare your new personal values with the values of your company. Do you think you will be able to stand by your personal values when you are at work? (Remember this is *key* for burnout prevention and recovery, so it's an important question to consider.)

Knowing the answers to these questions will help inform your decision-making about whether or not you can stay in your current job. We'll be making these decisions in Phase Three of the recovery process – for now, we're just thinking everything through.

Step 5: Exploring Work Possibilities

Once you have sufficiently restored your health (Step 3) and identified your new values (Step 4), the next step on the recovery journey is to explore the options available to you in the working world. This involves considering the changes you would want and/or need to make to return to your previous job (or to continue doing it if you haven't taken sick leave), as well as exploring new job opportunities, if that feels right for you. For example, you may have doubts about whether your employer will be able to make the adjustments you need to be able to work well. You might also be questioning whether your job really is right for you, now that you've reassessed your values. If this is the case, you will want to think about looking outside of your current work and consider alternative roles or organisations. You may even consider going self-employed or starting your own business.

The important thing at this stage is that you are only *thinking about* and *researching* possible changes and new opportunities without yet making decisions, actioning any of your options or committing to anything. It's crucial that you don't make any big career decisions this soon in your recovery journey – at this early stage, you must conserve what little energy you have for yourself. Take it slow. Step 5 is all about thinking, not doing.

If you're not sure where to start with exploring your job opportunities, keep reading, as I'll cover everything you need to know to work through Stage 5 now.

AM I READY FOR STEP 5?

I think it's important to ask if you're ready for Step 5 before we get going.

At this stage, if you have taken time off work, you need to be recovered enough to be able to discuss and explore with your employer reasonable adjustments for your return to work. For example, you need to be in a place where you'd feel comfortable contacting your line manager or HR department to discuss what adjustments you might need and hear what options they could make possible for you. You need to be comfortable with opening this dialogue so you can begin considering your options. If you've worked throughout your recovery, then opening these conversations about change with your employer can happen alongside your work.

If exploring your options feels OK to you then you are in the right part of your recovery journey to begin Step 5. However, if the thought of talking to your manager or HR department puts you into 'fight or flight' mode, you need to pull back and go back to restoring your health by revisiting the work in Phase One (Steps 1–3).

If you begin discussions with your employers but then find that you are getting really stressed when talking about changes at work, it's probably too early in your burnout recovery for you to go through this part of the process. In order to navigate this stage of recovery successfully, you must have improved regulation over your emotions before you can even consider beginning to contemplate and negotiate changes. If you're not there yet, you're not ready to reach this point. Again, I suggest you revisit Phase One (Steps 1–3) to focus on restoring your health. Make sure you take the time you need.

Coming to Terms With the Need to Make Changes

In my own burnout recovery I've been fortunate enough to have explored lots of different ways of making a post-burnout career work. The good news is that having a successful post-burnout career is absolutely possible, even if it looks and feels a little daunting right now!

There is no denying that your post-burnout career is likely to look very different to the previous hopes and aspirations you had for your career. This isn't necessarily a bad thing, as it could open up some incredible doors for you. That said, it's entirely normal to go through a period of bereavement and feeling sad for the career that you thought you would have.

Going through burnout and considering and making career changes is a bit like going through a rough patch in a long-term relationship, and deciding whether to stay or leave. When you first meet your partner, you love everything about them and throw yourself into the relationship – a bit like your career during the pre-burnout honeymoon phase (*see* p. 97). But then things start to get a bit stressful and the relationship becomes rocky, and eventually things are so bad that (despite having loved each other deeply) the harm inside the relationship comes to a head. A decision then has to be made about whether you stay together and work through the issues or whether you split. In your burnout recovery, this looks like the part where you start to consider whether you can stay in your current role that burned you out or whether it's time to leave.

This is a tough decision to make. At this stage in a relationship, you are likely to have worked hard and put a lot into it, and there might well still be some love there between you both. In the same way, you might still love your job despite it burning you out! But just as you can't stay in a relationship with someone who isn't willing to put the work in, or doesn't see how their behaviour is harmful, there comes a point in your burnout recovery when you need to work out if you can go back to your job and stay well or whether the workplace is just too toxic to remain. As midwife Leah Hazard explains:

> *Taking time off was not a luxury – it was absolutely essential to maintain any kind of functional quality of life. Then – and this is still an ongoing process – I left the area where I worked, and which I loved, for the last seven years, and decided to work clinically in other less-demanding roles. It's still tempting to return to where I was, but I know that staying away from that kind of excessive workload and psychologically unsafe environment is important for my ongoing recovery.*

Your employer might be able to make sufficient changes that could encourage you to stay and give things another go in your current job. However, just like in a relationship, when you might give it a second chance you could soon realise that the changes that have been offered aren't enough to keep you well and happy. You might find you still love your job or you might have fallen out of love with it, but either way it's not serving you, so you may feel it's time to move on.

If you do decide to leave your work then your future will be a different version of what you had hoped and planned for, and it's OK to feel sad about this. In the same way that when you commit to a relationship you will form a view of your incredible future together, you will have had the same for your career. Burnout and leaving your current role means saying goodbye to the future career you had planned for, and this can be emotionally challenging to navigate. Just like when a relationship ends, you will need to give yourself permission to grieve for what you thought you would get from your career.

Exploring Your Work Options

I have had the pleasure of advising many people about their post-burnout careers, and it's been brilliant to watch them flourish. As a result of this, I know that there is no single way to make your career work for you after burnout; you always have options and choices to consider. I am now going to give you the tools you need to explore these options and find your own path, regardless of what it is that you ultimately chose to do (as a reminder once again: this step is about exploring all options available to you rather than making actual decisions).

There are multiple work options available after burnout, but here is a broad overview:

- Returning to the same role in the same organisation
- Returning to a different role in the same organisation
- Returning to the same role in a different organisation
- Returning to a different role in a different organisation
- Going freelance/self-employed:
  - In the same sector
  - In a similar sector
  - In a completely different sector
- Creating a portfolio career (a career that consists of simultaneously having multiple part-time jobs, freelance projects or a business, often across various fields or industries)
- Starting and growing a business or becoming an entrepreneur

With so many options available, it would be impossible to cover all of them in a single book! Starting and growing a business, for instance, is a huge topic for which there are many fabulous resources already available for those that wish to pursue this direction.

With this in mind, I have chosen to focus on the following two areas:

1. **Returning to the same role in the same organisation (i.e. the role that burned you out):** This is important to discuss because I know that it will be the only option available to many people (whether that's on a temporary or permanent basis).
2. **Creating a portfolio career:** This way of working is the option that gives you the biggest amount of flexibility with the least amount of risk, but it is still very much the path less well trodden. That said, in my work as a career coach and mentor, this is probably the most popular option for people to explore post-burnout.

After we have discussed these two career options, I'll take you through writing a career development plan, which will help support you when it comes to making decisions about your career later on. I'll finish by sharing some common problems and mistakes made in this part of burnout recovery (so we can make sure that you avoid them!).

Option 1: Returning to the Same Role in the Same Organisation

Let's first look at how to return to the role that burned you out, and consider what tweaks can be made to help you stay well.

This option is worth considering, even if you don't see yourself in your current career long term. First, you might not be in a position to leave your current role (either financially or contractually), and second (and genuinely!), sometimes career satisfaction can be found simply by making some small tweaks to what you are currently doing.

To help you begin exploring the option of tweaking your current role, we'll be looking at the importance of job crafting.

Job Crafting

Job crafting means taking proactive steps to redesign what you do at work by changing the tasks you do, the relationships you have with colleagues and how you perceive your work. The idea of job crafting is to empower you to have control over your career which, as we learned in

Part I (*see* p. 41), is important because having a sense of control at work is brilliant protection against burnout.

There are three ways to job craft:

1. Task Crafting

This involves actively shaping and moulding your role, the tasks you do and the responsibilities that you have.

Changes you could make here might include giving preference to work tasks that suit your skills or interests, so that you are engaging with more 'meaningful work' (*see* box below) more of the time, rather than allowing your preferred tasks to always drop to the bottom of your to-do list.

For instance, if you enjoy mentoring junior colleagues, perhaps you could look to incorporate more of this type of work into your daily responsibilities. You could think about spending more time with your existing mentees or take on more mentees, if you have the time and capacity to do so.

It is important to recognise, however, that task crafting must happen within the parameters of your job description, and therefore there might be limitations as to how effectively you can craft your job (I go into this in a bit more detail on p. 156).

MEANINGFUL WORK: A REMINDER

As discussed in Part I (*see* p. 45), you actually only need to spend 20 per cent of your time doing personally meaningful work in order to reduce your burnout risk by half. This equates to one day out of a five-day working week, or one hour and forty minutes out of an average 8-hour working day. This is a manageable amount, which I believe we should all be aiming for and prioritising.

I've been asked previously: What does 'meaningful' work mean, exactly? The answer is that it's whatever work is meaningful to you. This means it's the work:

- that brings you the biggest satisfaction;
- that ignites the fire in your belly;

- that makes you the proudest and happiest;
- where you know you are making a big impact.

The idea here is to get you thinking about what tweaks could be made in your current job to ensure you spend more time (just 20 per cent!) doing the stuff that really excites you. It's all about being creative with how you work, and thinking about how you can delegate tasks or do them more efficiently in order to spend more time in your day doing the work you find meaningful.

To give an example, you might be a nurse and find that you are spending too much time doing paperwork rather than spending time with your patients or teaching nursing students, which is what you find personally meaningful. In this instance, you could perhaps look at how you could spend more time teaching students within the limitations of your current job description. Perhaps there could be more time for informal teaching at the bedside? Or maybe you could delegate some of the paperwork to someone else on the team?

Exercise 35

Make task crafting work for you
Complete Exercise 5 (p. 45) to work out what meaningful work means to you. Consider how you can tweak your current job role so that you end up doing meaningful work for 20 per cent of your time, and whether you need help to achieve this.

Think about:

- What can you tweak yourself within the current parameters of your job now?
- For bigger changes, who and what do you need help with to achieve this? For instance, you could consider setting up a meeting with HR to discuss options.

2. Relationship Crafting

Reshaping the nature of the interactions you have with others at work is called relationship crafting. Peer support and having a psychologically safe space at work has proven to be crucial post-burnout, and you can use relationship crafting to increase your social resources.

Changes you could make here might include:

- mentoring new employees;
- organising work social events;
- celebrating successes with colleagues;
- making friends with people who have similar skills or interests to you at work.

3. Cognitive Crafting

Cognitive crafting refers to how you can change your mindset about the tasks you do, i.e. reframing your thoughts about work to more positive ones. Changes you can make here might include reminding yourself of the importance of your work and how it positively impacts your life, and practising gratitude regularly.

For instance, you could reframe your attitude towards work from viewing it as simply completing tasks to thinking of these tasks as being integral to your company's success, by helping them with their mission and goals. You could shift your focus from the mundane or tedious aspects of the job to focusing on how your work has a positive impact on others (such as improving customer experience or supporting your colleagues). These simple reframes will shift your thinking about your job to be more helpful and positive – it really does make a difference!

The Benefits of Job Crafting

Job crafting can be very positive if you cannot leave your role or you're open to seeing if it can be improved with tweaks. In summary, it can help to:

- increase your level of engagement, happiness and meaning;
- increase your personal and professional growth;
- lead to better performance;
- lead to lower levels of sickness and burnout.

The Pitfalls of Job Crafting

There are some downsides to job crafting that we can't ignore. If your personal goals and values are misaligned with your employer's, you will struggle to job craft successfully.

Job crafting is also not an opportunity to change your job completely or beyond recognition. In order to job craft you have to have a job that can be altered, and some jobs are just more 'craftable' than others. Your seniority will likely affect how easy this process is, too.

As it is employee-initiated, there is a possibility that in job crafting you might take on too much, which could impact your recovery. This is a very real risk after burnout particularly, as a lot of people that burn out are high-achieving and conscientious.

Job crafting also risks exploitation by employers, if used incorrectly. The idea of job crafting is to empower the employee to have control over their career, but unfortunately I have seen it being used by some employers as an opportunity to get employees to take on more work. If this happens, your burnout recovery will be jeopardised.

That said, job crafting is still very helpful to try after burnout and, as we've discussed, there are multiple benefits. If done mindfully, it can be a helpful tool to develop and shape your career into one that you could love.

Exercise 36

Crafting your job role

Give the following exercise a go. Think about:

- how you could craft your current role into something more meaningful;
- how you could tweak your *tasks* at work, your *relationships* at work and how you *think about* your work.

Now, write down five positive statements about your work that will help to reframe your current thinking. If you find that your job is not easily craftable, then realising this now is a helpful part of the process as you think about the work opportunities available to you.

Option 2: Creating a Portfolio Career

The second work option we'll explore together is creating a portfolio career. A portfolio career is where you create your own unique career that consists of multiple part-time jobs or freelance projects or involves having a business simultaneously, often across various fields or industries.

Today, a job for life doesn't exist in the same way that it likely did for our parents. We live in a world where moving frequently between roles, industries, locations and careers is becoming the new normal, but that said, I'd say portfolio career working is still very much the career path less well trodden. However, it is becoming a more common way of working, and it can be an interesting (and exciting) option to explore post-burnout.

I've seen portfolio careers described as 'squiggly careers', and this description is pretty spot on. Each portfolio career is unique and it can be a really fun way of working. In practice, I have increasingly seen the medics I've helped with career coaching and mentoring choose to develop portfolio careers after burnout. This is because this way of working typically gives them a form of stability (by keeping their main line of work going with reduced hours), coupled with the freedom to explore whatever they want outside of their main line of work.

A portfolio career can be seen as the perfect way to balance risk as you're keeping as many options open as possible. It's also a helpful way to manage a transition to another job (whether that's within the same industry or not) or even to start a business.

I chose to pursue a portfolio career path after burnout. I've held multiple roles at different times alongside my GP work, including: being a Health Inequalities Fellow; doing a postgraduate certificate in public health; setting up my own aesthetics business; running a subscription box for medics; and working as a tutor for the University of Bristol Medical School. I then became an NHS clinical entrepreneur and started working on the thing that really puts fire in my belly: burnout prevention. (I would just add that I didn't do all of this at once...!)

I view my post-burnout career as an evolutionary process of trying new things and working out a way that I can make my career work for me. It has become a running joke among my friends and family that I collect and get offered jobs on a regular basis – but it has definitely been the right way of working for me after my burnout.

I do recognise, however, that I am extremely fortunate to be able to have this degree of flexibility with my career, and I know that this is a privilege that is not afforded to everyone. I also know that some contracts do not allow employees to have other work. That said, I do think exploring the opportunities around portfolio career working is still worth it, even if you work in an industry that doesn't typically allow for such flexibility. Find out what might be possible because portfolio career working has so many fabulous things to offer if you can make it work.

If you go down this portfolio route, you will find that opportunities come your way and doors will open up that you never even thought possible. It's a very exciting way to work, but you must be able to embrace the emotional rollercoaster and financial insecurity that it typically brings.

To create a portfolio career that works for you, you will need to develop the following: a clear understanding of your strengths and values; self-confidence to put yourself out there and ask for work; networks and relationships; and an ability to explore options and assess their possibilities. (The upcoming advice on how to write a career development plan will really help you if a portfolio career is something that you want to explore further, *see* p. 161.)

Benefits of a Portfolio Career

- You're never bored!
- You will have multiple opportunities to learn new skills.
- You will have increased autonomy and control over your career (which, as you know, is essential for both burnout prevention and recovery).
- You will have the flexibility to prevent and manage any current or future burnout by creating protected opportunities for rest.

- You will earn higher than average income (helpful to know, especially if you are worried about finances).
- If you're not able to leave the job that burned you out yet, a portfolio career could, in time, lead to more work choices (for example, you could ask to go to fewer days a week with your main job, and then spend the extra time focusing on an alternative career strand to begin).

Pitfalls of a Portfolio Career

- It's tiring and time-consuming to find and pursue new opportunities, especially when you're already exhausted after burnout.
- You can potentially take on too much in the excitement of being offered new opportunities; you must pace yourself after burnout!
- You need a large capacity for change and lots of flexibility, which might not be suitable for everyone.
- Your admin skills need to be next level, as having a portfolio career typically involves: having multiple email addresses, handling many contacts, proactively chasing invoices and payment, as well as lots of organisation in terms of arranging meetings and annual leave.
- Your financial and tax affairs are likely to become quite complicated and you will need an accountant.

How to Create a Portfolio Career

To help you explore the option of a portfolio career, these questions will get you thinking. (In addition, you can use the career development plan, on p. 161.) Consider the following in reference to a portfolio career and nailing down some initial ideas:

1. **Why do you want to have a portfolio career?** List all the positives and negatives that you can think of and then consider if this might be an option you'd like to explore further (if it's not,

that's still great information to have gathered!). If you feel that this is an option you'd like to explore further, move on to the next question.

2. **What are your diverse interests and skills?** Think about your interests and skills, beyond your current job. What interests do you have (either professional or personal) that you enjoy and are passionate about? List as many things as you can.

3. **How could you incorporate these interests and skills into your work life?** Consider freelance projects, part-time roles or hobbies that can generate income. Think outside the box – the great thing about having a portfolio career is that you have complete flexibility. For instance, if you currently work for a bank but fancy a portfolio career, there's nothing to stop you from setting up that side hustle in a creative industry that you've always fancied, alongside keeping some shifts in your old office, if that's an option.

4. **Can you visualise a balanced portfolio career?** Envision a life where you engage in multiple roles or projects. How would you structure your time and energy across these activities? Consider time management, financial stability and personal fulfilment and think about what you'd like your working week to look like. You'd need to ensure that you're not going to take on too much too soon after burnout.

Now it's time to think about the practical side of things. Consider the following:

1. **Is it viable?** Is there a need or a market for what you'd want to do?
2. **What are your networking connections?** Who would you need to speak to and connect with?
3. **How financially viable are your options?** Can you afford to do what you want to? If not, how could you work around this temporarily?
4. **What would you need to do to get started?**

Then move on to the next section to consider this further as we create a career development plan.

Writing a Career Development Plan

If you ask anyone what you should do with your career, the chances are they will come back with an idea that focuses on a specific role. But I want to encourage you to think about your career in an entirely different way after burnout, so to help with this I'm going to take you step by step through writing a career development plan.

From working through these steps, you should by now have an idea of what you want to achieve in terms of:

- what meaningful work means for you, and how you can get some more meaningful work into your current role (*see* p. 153);
- whether or not your current role is 'craftable' and, if so, how you can start to shape your current role into one that works for you (*see* p. 152);
- what your values are, and how to use them in your career decision-making (*see* p. 144).

Now, we're going to take this information and create a roadmap to help you get there, by writing a career development plan. There are five stages to this process. In this phase of burnout recovery, remember that you are simply *thinking* about changes, rather than actioning them, therefore we're going to write your career development plan in two parts.

The first part that follows asks you to do an assessment of your current situation, identify your desired endpoint and work out where the gaps are in terms of skills, knowledge and qualifications. In Phase Three we'll work through the second part of the development plan with some decision-making and goal setting. (This second part of writing your career development plan is on p. 174 if you want to complete it all in one go.)

1. Assess Your Current Situation

Start by performing an analysis of where you're currently at by asking yourself the following:

- What do you enjoy about your job? What don't you enjoy?
- Which of your values are in alignment with your current job? Which aren't?
- Who and what inspires you in your current role?
- If you carry on this current path, where will you be in two years', five years' and ten years' time? Is this what you want?

2. Identify Your Desired Endpoint

We often think of the end goal in our careers as a job position or role, such as a CEO or lawyer. But the aim of this exercise is to let go of the traditional assumption of what our career endpoints 'should' be, and to focus instead on how you *want to* work, live, experience and feel in your career. You can use the two exercises below to help you explore this.

Exercise 37

Your dream career

Grab some paper, a pen and a cup of tea or glass of wine (if that's what you want). Sit down and intensely journal about your dream career and life. You are creating your fantasy life, so go wild. You have permission to write down extraordinary things that you feel might not be achievable.

You need to identify how you live and how you engage with your work, and you want to include *all* the detail. Outline every moment of your day, from when you wake up – what sort of house do you live in? Where is the house? Who is in the house with you? What are you eating for breakfast? What time are you eating breakfast? How are you getting to work? What car do you drive? What time do you arrive to work? What tasks are you doing at work? – to the moment you go to sleep. Include both weekdays and weekends.

You must cover your work day in detail – what tasks do you do? How much responsibility do you have? Who are you working for? What is your salary? What additional benefits might you have? What days or shift patterns do you work?

You must also cover your home lifestyle in detail – what do you do in your spare time? What hobbies do you have? What books are you reading? Where do you travel? What sort of property do you live in and do you own or rent it? Who is living with you at home? Are you single or married? Do you have children?

While you're doing this exercise, ask yourself how it would *feel* to live this life. I want you to experience the joy, the excitement and the hope.

Once you've completed your dream career exercise, the next step is to focus down your broad overall dream into something a little more focused in terms of a job role or plan with the following *ikigai* exercise. *Ikigai* is a Japanese concept that translates as 'reason for being'. Working out your *ikigai* basically means working out your career sweet spot.

Your *ikigai* is the feeling you get when what you enjoy doing, what the world needs, what you can be paid for and what you're good at all converge. If you're off balance with any one of these factors, you're going to feel off-kilter and a bit stuck.

If you're doing something that you love and what the world needs but you're not being paid very much, you're likely to feel fulfilled but (unless you have other sources of income or financial support) you'll be stressed about the bills. Another example would be if you're doing something that you can be paid for, it's what the world needs, and you're good at it, but you don't love it. In this scenario, you're going to feel financially comfortable, but unfulfilled.

Exercise 38

Your ikigai
Think about your *ikigai*:

- **What do you enjoy doing?** Write down every activity you enjoy and everything that sets your heart on fire.
- **What are you good at?** Write down every skill, attribute and qualification you have. Focus on your many strengths.
- **What can you get paid for?** Focus on what you can be paid for with your current skills and qualifications, but also how you could diversify.
- **What does the world need?** This is about what 'meaningful work' is for you. (Refer back to the meaningful work exercise for inspiration on p. 45, if helpful.) What work aligns with your values?

3. Perform a Gap Analysis

Now that you have an idea about your current situation (stage 1 of the career development plan) and your desired career end point (stage 2), we can perform a gap analysis. The aim here is to work out the gaps so that you can focus on filling them in to move you forward.

You need to acknowledge where you are now and then identify the skills, knowledge, help, experience and contacts you need so you can move forward towards your desired career end point. Think about:

- What skills and knowledge do you need to get to your desired end point?
- Do you need any additional skills?
- What help do you need?
- What experience do you need?
- Who do you need to help you?

Congratulations! You have now written the first part of your career development plan.

We're not yet going to make any decisions or put anything into action right now, as this stage of burnout recovery is simply about exploring your options, entirely free of the burden of having to make a choice. Therefore, feel free to write as many development plans as you wish for all the different career options that you want to explore. Play around with it and have fun – remember that this stage of recovery is about exploring as many options as possible, without committing to anything just yet. This is all wonderful groundwork for then going on to actively make decisions and commit to action in Phase Three of recovery.

Common Mistakes with Post-Burnout Career Development

When it comes to exploring career options in Phase Two, I see the same mistakes being made over and over again by people with burnout. (I've absolutely fallen foul of some of these pitfalls, as well.)

If you map out your ideas for your future career using the career development plan outlined above, then hopefully you'll avoid most of these mistakes. That being said, I think it's still helpful for you to be aware of the most common mistakes made after burnout, so you have the opportunity to avoid them.

1. Entering an Internet Spiral

Repeatedly googling 'alternative careers for X' (in my case, being a doctor) and falling into an internet spiral is something to avoid. (Hands up if you've done this yourself!) Google can be a good place to start when thinking about career options, but it becomes problematic when it's repeatedly turned to without any resolution or used in a scattergun fashion.

When using a search engine you'll get an awful lot of ideas, but in burnout your capacity for processing a lot of information is reduced, as is your decision-making ability. While searching the internet might appear to be making your life easier when exploring career opportunities, it's quickly going to become overwhelming.

2. Asking the Wrong Questions

There is nothing wrong with asking your peers for career advice, and networking is crucial for helping you make career decisions and for finding career opportunities. However, in order to get helpful answers, you must ask the *correct questions* of the *correct people* in the *correct setting*.

As an example, if you ask an internet forum a question such as, 'I'm having a horrific time at work, what shall I do next with my career?' you will get a whole stream of ideas come back to you, but *none* of these will be tailored to *you*, your circumstances or your wishes and preferences. The advice you get will be biased and based on the life experiences of others, which is likely to be coming from a good place but it doesn't necessarily mean that it's the right advice for you.

I see this all the time in medicine. For example, someone very junior might ask for advice because they're not enjoying the job, but they'll be told to get to the next stage of doctor training before deciding what to do next. This is almost always the advice, and it ignores the fact that the problems affecting the person asking the question are not necessarily going to disappear at the next stage of training. Without doubt, as you become more senior in medicine, things do change and the way you work changes. It might be that getting to the next stage of career progression *will* make everything better, and we can all tolerate some temporary discomfort if that's the case. But, actually, if the things that are not right about the job for you are still going to be present – or perhaps even worse – at senior levels, then sticking it out is bad advice.

The other issue with asking peers or colleagues for advice is confirmation bias. This occurs when you only see your immediate colleagues or network doing the same thing with their careers. This then leads you to think that the only career options available to you are the ones that you can see, or know that others are doing. The truth is, there are so many incredible options out there. The best way to overcome this is to network and surround yourself with people who are exploring other ways of working, beyond those who are immediately in front of you.

When speaking to other people for career advice, simply be curious. Ask lots of questions about how and why others have ended up in the careers they have, and what the good and the not so good aspects of it are. Then you can consider if what they've done might be a good fit for you.

3. Thinking Any Job Would be Better Than Your Current Role

The next common career mistake I see after burnout is thinking that *anything* is better than what you currently have, so applying for positions without really considering if they are the best fit for you. You'd be surprised at how often I see this.

I previously held a fellowship post, and during this time the organisation I was working for was advertising a new post. One of my friends was leading the interviews, and was shocked that about half of the candidates when asked, 'Why do you want this job?' said, 'I don't like my current job and I'm looking to do anything else.'

Essentially, they were not adequately researching the role and were blindly applying in the hope of getting something different to what they already had. Unsurprisingly, none of these candidates got the job. I totally understand the desperation to move on and get out of a difficult job because of burnout, but please – don't be that person!

4. Expecting a New Role to Solve Your Problems

The above ties in nicely to another mistake people often make: thinking that achieving a certain job role or status will fix things. Taking on more seniority or a different role won't automatically solve your problems; it all depends on what your problems are in the workplace.

5. Not Having Realistic Expectations About Your Capacity for Work

A final, very common career mistake after burnout is not having realistic expectations about your capacity for work. While having burnout doesn't mean that you can never work again, or that you cannot work full-time, it does change your capacity for work – at least temporarily. This is incredibly hard to come to terms with, especially for the type-A driven, overachieving type that typically burns out.

When you are in this particular phase, you will not yet be fully recovered (remember, complete recovery can take years). Therefore, you are likely to have ongoing difficulties with symptoms such as fatigue for some time to come. This is all totally normal and part of the process, but you must make changes to your work life that recognise this new normal for you.

You must have realistic expectations about how much energy you will have for work from now on, and how much rest you will need. Things *do* get easier the further away from your burnout that you move, but when you return to work (or when you are so close to your burnout, if you are still working) you will need some adjustments made to allow you to remain well. Burnout will affect your stamina, emotional resilience, and mental and emotional capacity. You must be kind and gentle with yourself, as this part of burnout recovery can be equally frustrating and distressing.

Exercise 39

Learn from your mistakes
Think about:

- Have you made any of these common mistakes in the past?
- How can you be sure to avoid them in the future?

How to Know When Phase Two is Complete

Phase Two is all about preparing for change, whether you are staying in the role that burned you out or deciding you are going to move on and explore new possibilities.

You are ready to move on to enact these changes when:

- you are still well (Step 3);
- you've picked your five values from the list on p. 145 and feel happy and confident with your choices (Step 4);
- you now have ideas about the options available to you, and you will have started to explore lots of different career ideas for the future (Step 5).

If you find that you are not well, or if you have not completed Steps 4 or 5, please go back for now and do this work first. I encourage you to wait until you are genuinely ready to move on, and do not pressure yourself to go further ahead before you are ready. The next stage of recovery is Phase Three, where you will actually be making decisions and then taking action, so you need to be ready for this.

PHASE THREE: ACTIONING CHANGE

You're now at the point in your burnout recovery journey where – hopefully – you've restored your health (Steps 1–3), revised your values (Step 4) and explored your career options (Step 5). Huge congratulations, because this is *hard*! (If you're not at this point yet, hang on in there; continue to do the work and come back to this section when you're ready.)

Burnout recovery takes on average one to three years, and when you are thinking about a return to work or making changes, you have not likely taken anywhere near that length of time off. You will not yet fully be recovered and won't be for a while. Particularly in the early days, you will still have a lower threshold for feeling stressed and anxious and your fatigue is also likely to be overwhelming. Therefore, this phase will be a very vulnerable time for you – you must continue to respect your burnout and have realistic expectations of yourself and others as you navigate your work and life changes.

Now, we move on to the third phase of burnout recovery, which is taking action. Calling this the final stage of recovery is, I believe, a bit of a misnomer, because making a change isn't the end of your burnout journey; it's simply the start of another chapter of post-burnout life where all decisions must respect your burnout. Going back to work after burnout means making considerable changes, having the strength to maintain these changes and managing any resistance to changes at an individual, team and organisational level, as well as ensuring that you stay well physically and emotionally. I'll guide you through the processes of identifying exactly which changes to go for, how to successfully implement them and how to maintain these changes for your continued health and a sustained recovery. Let's get started with Step 6.

Step 6: Making Changes at Work

Step 6 is all about making effective changes and taking action to stop yourself from burning out again. In this step, we will touch on how to decide which changes to make (from the options you explored in Step 5), how to return well to work (if you have taken time off sick), and how to implement your boundaries at work in order to sustain your recovery.

The action part of making change can be broken down into the following parts:

1. Deciding on change
2. Implementing change
3. Maintaining change

1. Deciding on Change

Now it's crunch time: time to decide your next career steps. Having gone through Phase Two of the recovery process, you will have done your research and will know which career options and changes are available to you. Regardless of whether you've taken sick leave or not, you will have been in discussion with your work about which changes they can support you with (and which ones they cannot), and you will have done your own deep dive into what it is that you might want for yourself, too.

It's now time to bite the bullet and make some decisions. I want to help you through this process because I understand how tricky making decisions about your post-burnout career can feel. I know from my own personal experience that you are likely to worry that making a wrong decision may inadvertently cause you to slip back into burnout. I can't promise that you won't make mistakes along the way, but if you are able to make decisions about your future in alignment with your new post-burnout values (as we'll discuss next), then the chances of you stalling or jeopardising your hard-won progress will be vastly reduced.

TRY NOT TO JUDGE YOURSELF

Don't beat yourself up for decisions that you have made in the past when your values might have been different. Regardless of the consequences of any prior decision-making, remember that those decisions were made in good faith with the tools and information that you had at the time.

Also remember to hold yourself with compassion if the decisions you make now don't work out in the future. If this happens, simply take stock, consider your options again and use your values to help you make further decisions.

It's time to begin making decisions. So, grab your list of values and your career development plan from Phase Two, and read on. (If you haven't done this work yet, revisit Phase Two and come back when it's done.)

Value-Based Decision-Making

When you're contemplating any big decision (regardless of whether it's about your post-burnout career or not), if you go back to your values (*see* p. 145) you really can't go wrong. This is true for any type of decision, whether your options are limited or unwanted, or you have multiple choices and are finding it hard to narrow them down. If you always go back to your guiding principles (i.e. your values), you know that you are making the decision that is right for you at this present time.

Post-burnout, you will often have to make some difficult choices, so use the questions below to help guide you to a values-based decision. I recommend carving out some protected time in your diary to do this:

- What decision are you considering?
- What are your options?
- How do your options align with your values?
- How do your options conflict with your values?
- What are your red lines?
- Which value(s) do you have to absolutely honour?

- Which value(s) are you willing to compromise?
- Based on your previous answers, which decision is the best fit for your values? Why?

If you're facing a big decision and there are two or more options that align with your values, you might consider writing a list of pros and cons, but this won't always move you on or be helpful. If writing a list of pros and cons isn't sufficient, ask the question again but flip it to be the *opposite* of the original. For instance, if the first question was, 'What are the pros and cons of taking this new job?' ask yourself, 'What are the pros and cons of *not* taking this new job?' Reframing the question will allow you to explore some nuances that might help you to make that important choice.

Exercise 40

Using value-based questions
Now use the value-based questions above to make decisions on the following:

- Are you going to continue in the same job that burned you out or are you going to leave?
- If you are going to continue, what accommodations are you going to ask for?
- If you are going to leave, what are you going to do next and how are you going to achieve this?

2. Implementing Change

Once you have made a decision about what you are going to do next in your recovery (now would be the perfect time to revisit your workplace/individual risk factors, *see* p. 39), it's time to implement those changes. To help you do this well, I am going to take you through the following:

- Finishing your career development plan
- How to return to work well after sick leave
- Boundary setting

Finishing Your Career Development Plan

Grab the career development plan that you started to write in Phase Two (*see* p. 161). (*see* p. 161) Now you've made a decision about your next steps, we're going to help you successfully make change by setting goals and writing an action plan to support your decision by implementing changes.

SMARTR goal setting

You've most likely heard of SMART goals, but I like to add on an 'R' for 'rewarded' because, generally, I think we can be really terrible at rewarding ourselves when we achieve our goals. After burnout, celebrating the wins and really leaning into the happiness that they bring is crucial after a period of feeling despondent for so long. (Also, in rewarding ourselves, we are helping our brain to positively reinforce behaviour changes, which makes us more likely to continue with good habits and goal achievement.) So, let me introduce you to a SMARTR goal:

Specific
Measurable
Achievable
Realistic
Time bound
Rewarded

I'm going to give you a fictional example here to help you visualise what a non-SMARTR goal and a SMARTR goal look like in practice. Let's imagine a burned-out lawyer that has decided to leave law behind and set up a floristry business. They can't leave their job entirely just yet because they still need to bring in a wage due to their financial responsibilities. The lawyer's employer has already agreed to them going part-time.

An example of a non-SMARTR goal here would be: 'I want to reduce my hours as a lawyer and start a floristry business.'

This goal – while a great thing to aspire to – isn't going to help the lawyer get to where they want to be. First, it's not clear exactly what they mean by reducing their hours, and the strategy for starting their new business is also unclear. There is no time frame associated with the goal either, so no deadline of which the person setting this goal will be motivated to hit.

If you wanted to make this goal SMARTR, you might say something like this: 'I want to transition from a full-time legal career to a flourishing floristry business within one year, while maintaining part-time legal work.' Let's dig into the detail of this lawyer's SMARTR goal to discuss each component:

Specific: I will reduce my full-time hours as a lawyer to part-time (20 hours per week) and dedicate at least 20 hours per week to developing and launching my floristry business.

Measurable: I will reduce my legal work hours to 20 per week by the end of the first month; complete a comprehensive business plan for the floristry business within the first two months; launch a basic version of the floristry business (including website and social media presence) within six months; and secure at least five regular clients and generate a minimum monthly income of £2,000 from floristry by the end of the first year.

Achievable: I will use my part-time legal income to support my personal expenses and my savings will fund the initial business costs. I will also attend floristry workshops and network with local businesses to build skills and connections.

Realistic: The goal set allows me to move away from a stressful legal career in sequential steps that are realistic for my current energy levels and capacity, while not causing any unnecessary financial stress.

Time-bound: I will reduce legal hours to part-time within a month; complete the business plan within two months; launch the floristry business within six months and achieve my financial goals from the floristry business within the first year.

Rewarded: On getting my first client, I will celebrate by buying an affordable piece of art for the wall of my new floristry studio. (Your rewards don't have to cost much – or any – money; sometimes achieving the goal is inherently rewarding in itself. If you would like to mark it, your reward could be meeting a friend for a walk or buying something small like a book or nail polish. However, if you choose to reward yourself, savour it and remind yourself why you're doing it.)

While this example is fictional, hopefully it is obvious that succeeding at achieving the SMARTR goal is far more likely than achieving the non-SMARTR goal, as the SMARTR goal has been carefully considered and mapped out in detail.

ACT SMART

An alternative option if you are a recovering people pleaser or perfectionist (*see* p. 69) might be to try the ACT approach to SMART goals, which is slightly different and can sometimes feel more accessible. SMART goals in ACT look like:

Specific actions
Motivated by values/meaningful
Adaptive
Realistic
Time framed

As you can see, S, R and T are the same as in traditional SMART goals. There is no additional R in ACT SMART goals. However:

M asks you to take actions that are motivated by values or that are meaningful to you. I've already covered how important it is to make sure that you bear your values in mind when making post-burnout decisions (*see* p. 141), and the ACT approach to SMART goals embeds this into the process.

A is adaptive rather than achievable. Adaptive means answering the question: 'Is this wise?' It asks you to look at the bigger picture and ask yourself if your decision will mean that your life will be better in the long run. Is the right thing to be setting, given your current resources and capacity?

Exercise 41

Writing your SMARTR goal

Write a single* SMARTR goal to support the decision you have made for your future career direction.

I recommend writing a single sentence that states your overall goal, and then to write short paragraphs that detail each individual element – just as I demonstrated with our fictional lawyer above. Flick back to p. 174 for a reminder of how I did this, and feel free to use that structure to write your single SMARTR goal.

* Please note: you are welcome to write more than one SMARTR goal, but after burnout I recommend keeping your goals to a minimum for ease (and an increased chance of success) as you recover.

Write An Action Plan for Your SMARTR goal

Now you have your SMARTR goal outlined, the next thing to do is to write your action plan. Your action plan is going to help you stay on track to achieve your goal, by breaking down the process into manageable steps, and by scheduling regular reviews and evaluation of your progress. Your action plan would typically include:

- identifying specific tasks;
- setting timelines;
- allocating resources;
- establishing checkpoints to monitor progress.

This is a really helpful framework, but do remember that – regardless of which version of SMARTR goals that you chose to use to create your action plan – you must respect your burnout when it comes to timeframes and how quickly you wish to achieve your goals. You *must* make sure that you factor in adequate rest time, and allow for the fact that it will most likely take you longer to achieve your goals than pre-burnout. Don't set yourself up for failure from the start; it's better to give yourself too much time than too little.

Here's what the action plan for our burned-out lawyer might look like:

Month 1: Begin the reduction in hours with the current legal employer. Research and enrol in floristry courses to enhance skills.

Month 2: Write a detailed business plan for the floristry business. Identify and contact potential suppliers for flowers and materials.

Months 3–4: Develop a brand identity (name, logo and business cards). Create a website and set up social media accounts.

Months 5–6: Start marketing the floristry business through social media and local advertisements. Network with local event planners and businesses for potential partnerships.

Months 7–12: Focus on securing clients through excellent service and word of mouth. Monitor finances and adjust strategies to meet financial goals. Continue professional development in floristry and business management.

Evaluate your goals at the following intervals:

Monthly check-ins: Review progress on reducing legal work hours, business plan development and floristry skills improvement. Review current work-life balance and any change to stress levels or burnout symptoms.

Quarterly reviews: Assess business launch progress, client acquisition and income generation.

Annual evaluation: Determine success in transitioning to floristry, achieving income goals and overall work-life satisfaction. Adjust future goals as needed based on this evaluation.

Remember that, in this example, our lawyer's goal is to have established their floristry business within a year, so the action plan reflects this timeline. However, you have total flexibility about your own time frame, and you can chose to move more quickly, or slowly, depending on what your goal is. If you achieve your goal quickly, don't forget to come back and set another! This process will set you up for success, regardless of what your goal is or where you are in your burnout.

Exercise 42

Write your own action plan
Use the example action plan above to help write your own action plan. Add the reviews for the evaluation process into your diary now.

Now, select one thing to work towards this week to get the process of achieving your goal started!

How to Return to Work Well After Sick Leave

If you have been off sick with burnout, now is the time that you'll be heading back into the workplace. (If you haven't taken sick leave, feel free to skip past this section, but I do suggest you read the box on advocating for yourself after burnout, *see* p. 181.)

Having a sense of control over your work life and maintaining good relationships is key for a successful recovery at this stage, so this is what you need to prioritise when negotiating and making decisions about the detail of your return to work.

This is important because if you go back into the exact circumstance that burned you out, you will burn out again – there is no doubt about it. Even if you are starting to feel better after a period of sick leave, you are likely to still be in a position of considerable emotional vulnerability. This, coupled with the physical fatigue of having burnout, means that you will have a reduced capacity for asking for change at work when you return, so I want to share these tips with you now.

1. **Open a two-way dialogue with your manager** in good time before you go back to work. They will be able to suggest reasonable adjustments to help you when you return. This might include increased supervision, protected rest time, going back part-time with a view to increasing your hours, and amended duties. Your

requirements will be unique to you and your circumstances, so now is the time to decide on what feels right.

2. **Your doctor can write a sick note** with reasonable adjustments outlined. (If you need help with this, don't forget that your doctor can always advocate for you and support your return to work as well.)

3. **Have reasonable expectations** as to how and what your employer can change for you at work. They will have obligations and expectations as well, and it might be that the things that you would like to have changed are not going to be achievable. What's really important is that you have *some* change and that you feel you have a sense of control and autonomy over those changes.

4. **Being treated with kindness and being part of a supportive team** makes all the difference when you go back to work after sick leave. If you have difficulties with an individual, that doesn't necessarily mean that you can't return to work. The key thing here is to ask who the majority of your interactions will be with, how that will affect you, and what you can reasonably do about it. For example, if you're coming up against one individual that's causing problems, you might be able to report this to someone else. Escalate internally if that is the case to see how your organisation might respond.

5. **Ensure that your new post-burnout values are in alignment with your organisation's values**. We've talked about the importance of identifying your values and engaging with values-based decision-making already (*see* pp. 141–47). Even if you're coming up against a little resistance or difficulty, if you feel that your values are generally in alignment with your organisation, this can sometimes be sufficient to help you through the difficult times.

6. **Try some self-directed changes**, if your organisation is finding it hard to make changes for you (*see* p. 54). Tweaking your role and adding in some more meaningful work will help.

7. **Start looking for work elsewhere** if your requests for change are reasonable, but you're coming up against resistance; if the organisational culture doesn't align with your new values at all; or if the whole working culture feels toxic.

8. **Ensure that you are well supported when you return**, both inside and outside of work. Remember to treat yourself with kindness and self-compassion as you adjust to your new post-burnout normality. I recommend regular review schedules with your manager or HR to review your situation, as everyone's recovery is different and you're likely to have to make continual adjustments as you go through your return to work.

HOW TO EFFECTIVELY ADVOCATE FOR YOURSELF AT WORK AFTER BURNOUT

Burnout is a vulnerable time. It can feel intimidating to ask for what you need – and never more so than when you run the risk of a negative response. If you are finding it difficult to ask for the changes you need at work because of pressure from your managers, the expectations of your colleagues or because you just don't know how to go about doing it, then here is my guide to help empower you to ask for the changes you need in burnout when it feels hard.

The Ashley ABCDEF on how to advocate for yourself in burnout

Ask for change, but propose a solution. Going to your line manager with solutions rather than problems will ultimately be better received. (A also stands for *audit trail* – make sure you get any agreed changes in writing. This is both to protect you and to make sure that your employer is held accountable.)

Be in a group. Asking for changes collectively often feels safer and will carry more weight behind it. There is strength in numbers. (B also stands for *believing you are worthy of change*. One of the barriers to successful advocacy is self-blame. If you are finding things stressful at work because of factors outside of your control, please recognise that it isn't all you. The guilt really does a number on us all.)

Care. Get support from your peers and from your loved ones outside of work.

Debrief. Ask for measurable outcomes and planned reviews of the changes and outcomes with your employer. This debrief exercise helps with accountability.

Energy. Respect your burnout. If you are early on in your recovery or if your burnout scores are high, save your energy for yourself and be selective about the battles you pick. It might be easier in the moment to choose the low-hanging fruit (the things that are easy to change) until you feel well enough to tackle the bigger stuff.

F*ck it! The worst that can happen is they say no. Truthfully, if they treat you poorly, that will make your career and life decision-making much easier.

Boundary Setting

The final part of how to successfully implement change at work, which is relevant regardless of which changes you chose to make, is all about setting and implementing your professional boundaries.

Boundary setting is an effective way of getting control back at work. Control (or a lack of it), as you now know, is one of the workplace factors that causes burnout in the first place, and knowing you are in control at work is one of the predictors of a successful recovery. So, as you action changes at work, your boundaries will be important.

Quite often in the slide into burnout, boundaries get pushed, lost and eventually obliterated. It's all too easy to fall into a cycle of people pleasing and overworking, where we lose that sense of what we can realistically take on. Worse, in professions where burnout is a common issue, the systems of working often make it challenging to put effective boundaries in place – and to maintain them.

There are boundary pushers everywhere. Your colleagues and your peers will push your boundaries. The system you work in will push your boundaries. You are the only person therefore that can maintain your boundaries, and when you're feeling burned out this can feel like a huge thing to tackle successfully. But, it can be done!

There are seven types of boundaries:

1. **Physical** – protecting your physical space and your body.
2. **Sexual** – protecting your right to consent and levels of intimacy.
3. **Emotional/mental** – protecting your right to have your own feelings and thoughts and to not have them criticised or invalidated.
4. **Spiritual** – protecting your right to worship as you wish, and practise your spiritual or religious beliefs.
5. **Intellectual** – protecting your thoughts and ideas.
6. **Financial/material** – protecting your financial resources and possessions.
7. **Time** – protecting how you spend your time.

For the purposes of this book, we will be focusing on your boundaries as they come into play at work, but what you learn here will help you in all aspects of your life. Let's start the journey to healthier boundaries by first assessing how healthy your boundaries are currently with the following exercise.

Exercise 43

How healthy are your boundaries?
Answer the yes/no questions below. Keep a note of your answers as we'll tally them up at the end.

1. Do you often feel overwhelmed by the demands and expectations of others?
2. Do you frequently put other people's needs before your own?

3. Do you find it difficult to say 'no', even when you are already stretched thin?
4. Do you feel guilty or anxious when you take time for yourself?
5. Do you often work beyond your regular hours or take on additional tasks without extra compensation?
6. Do you regularly experience physical symptoms of stress, such as headaches or fatigue, due to overcommitment?
7. Do you find yourself frequently apologising for things that are not your fault or beyond your control?
8. Do you feel responsible for other people's feelings and problems?
9. Do you struggle to delegate tasks, even when you are overwhelmed?
10. Do you often neglect your personal interests and hobbies due to work or obligations to others?

Now let's interpret your scores. Where do you fit with the following? Count the number of yes answers given:

0–2: You have relatively healthy boundaries.

3–5: How you recognise and implement your boundaries would benefit from some improvements; consider addressing areas where you feel the most pressure.

6–10: You have poor boundaries, which are likely to be contributing significantly to your burnout and might hinder an effective recovery. It's important to seek support and develop strategies to establish healthier boundaries.

The fewer yes answers selected, the healthier your boundaries are. But don't worry if you have more yeses than noes because I will help you start to redress some of the imbalance now.

To begin working on your boundaries we must first work out where your boundaries lie, and how and when they are being pushed. We can begin this through the exercise opposite.

Exercise 44

Where are your boundaries being pushed?

Think of all the times you've said yes to something where you wish you'd said no or when you've agreed to something then felt resentful or angry at yourself for saying yes. Follow the resentment – this is where your boundaries sit.

Write down as many examples of this as you can remember, then assess your list and take stock:

- What types of requests have triggered this type of response?
- What is the typical context of the request?
- Are there any common themes or patterns you can identify?

For instance, you might find that the requests that make you feel angry are the urgent ones that come towards the end of the day, when you're already swamped with work and know that you're likely to be staying late to finish your tasks. Or, it might be that you are consistently asked to perform tasks outside of your job description.

How to Push Back Respectfully?

Once you have an idea of the situations and circumstances that cause your boundaries to be pushed, the next thing to think about is how to push back against these unreasonable requests. (Remember, boundary setting isn't about shying away from doing work that you are ultimately responsible for, or making life difficult for anyone else. Instead, it's simply about correcting the imbalances that led to your burnout.)

To asset your boundaries, it's helpful to have some sentences in your arsenal that you can fire out when you're put on the spot. We can probably all identify with something happening and afterwards thinking, 'Oh, I wish I'd said something different!', then beating ourselves up for not being more assertive or communicating more effectively in the moment.

Let's try to break this cycle! Here are three suggestions for pushing back:

1. Simply Saying No

Remember that 'no' is a complete sentence. You don't have to give anyone an explanation about why you're pushing back on a certain boundary. A simple 'no' or 'no, I can't, unfortunately' will suffice in asserting yourself.

For those of us who are people pleasers and caregivers (I am a fully paid-up member of this club myself), I think that saying no on its own is really hard to do. In fact, sometimes there are challenging circumstances when you can't say no for whatever reason, be it the nature of your work, your gender, your race or your socio-economic circumstances. In this instance, you can try one of the following options....

2. Using a Pause

It might be more comfortable for you to set the boundary with a pause, rather than saying no.

Let me share an example to explain what I mean. A doctor local to me had a horrible episode of burnout. On coming back to work after a period of sick leave, their response to any question that was asked of them that pushed their boundaries was, 'Let me think about that.' This is a really good phrase because it says to the person asking the question: 'I've heard what you've said and I'm going to take some time to consider my response before getting back to you.' Alternative phrases for introducing a pause include: 'I need some time to think about it' or 'I'll come back to you.' Play around with what feels right for you.

If the request is not time sensitive, then a pause is a helpful way to delay the decision until you can come up with a way of articulating your response in a way that you're comfortable with (i.e. not having to answer on the spot).

3. Offering Alternative Solutions

Another technique to soften the blow of saying no is to offer up alternative solution. For example, you can signpost the person to other people or resources that can help. You could say something like, 'I'd love to help with that, but I can't right now. Can I suggest that you speak to someone else [and you can name them here]?' Or you could say, 'Come back to me in [a certain amount of time] when I should have more time to be able to help you.'

Learning to effectively implement your boundaries in burnout likely won't be a straightforward process, because you will get inevitable push back at some point. This can be extremely challenging to deal with, especially while you are still recovering. It takes courage to stand up for yourself, especially after burnout, so hold yourself with kindness and compassion.

I learned the hard way that holding my professional boundaries is essential for my mental well-being and continued ability to work. I figure that I can have more impact and do better things for others by being able to work. Think of your boundaries as an essential standard that you set for yourself – and you deserve the highest standards.

Exercise 45

Prevent your boundaries from being pushed

Be at the ready to push back against unreasonable requests.

1. Write down a 'no' sentence that you can easily memorise and use if your boundaries are challenged.
2. Write down a 'pause' sentence that you can easily memorise and use if your boundaries are challenged but you need to buy yourself some time.
3. Write down an 'alternative solution' sentence that you can easily memorise and use if your boundaries are challenged and you want to divert the request elsewhere.

The next time a boundary is pushed, commit to using one of these sentences!

3. Maintaining Change

It's now time to focus on making the hard-fought-for changes stick. This is essential so that you can continue to progress in your recovery.

The Seven Rs for Lasting Change

You'll have made significant changes to how you live, work and cope with your stress after burnout. You now need to work to sustain this. The disappointing truth is that it's really hard to make any behaviour changes stick. Just look at the huge numbers of bestselling books on behaviour change, the thousands of productivity apps and millions of views of habit hack videos available on social media. If it were that easy to undo years and years of engrained and learned behaviour, we'd all be doing it and there wouldn't be such an appetite for behaviour change support.

However, I'll be sharing with you now the seven Rs, which are practical strategies for making those crucial changes *genuinely* last. Even better, it doesn't have to mean getting up at 5am to work on your productivity and well-being when you'd far rather be asleep (unless, of course, that's what you want to do, in alignment with your values).

The seven Rs are: reminders, records, rewards, routines, relationships, reflecting and restructuring. These tips are easily accessible to all. Let's go through each one in turn.

1. Reminders

I don't know about you, but I lead a very busy life juggling work and family responsibilities and I often feel like my brain is like a computer with far too many tabs open. Reminding and prompting ourselves to engage in any new behaviour can be tricky, even when you're highly motivated to make change. But without doing the new behaviour regularly it will never become a habit, so it's important to find a way to remind yourself to do it regularly.

How you remind yourself to stick to your new behaviour is entirely up to you; the only caveat is that it's easy to do and fits in with your lifestyle. You could use the old favourite of writing a message on a card and sticking it on the fridge, propping it against the bathroom mirror or taping it to the car dashboard. Or write something in your diary, calendar or in the Notes app of your smartphone. You could just use one word, like 'breathe' or 'pause', and have it set as an alarm on your phone. Whatever it takes to remind you to do the new behaviour, do it repeatedly and consistently.

2. Records

Keeping a record of your behaviour by journaling or using a habit tracker is helpful for accountability. If you chose to journal, you just need five minutes at the end of the day to note down when and where you did the new behaviour and what the benefits were. (It's also helpful to write down when and where you do the old behaviour and what the costs/negative impacts are.)

Any diary or notebook – on paper or on-screen – works. Alternatively, there are many habit tracker apps available to download to help you track your goals and habits.

3. Rewards

It's important to reward yourself when you stick to new behaviours. Hopefully any new behaviour that involves acting on our values should be rewarding in its own right and you might not need anything further; however, additional rewards can help to reinforce it.

These rewards don't necessarily need to be expensive. One form of reward is kind, encouraging self-talk, for example saying to yourself: 'Well done, you did it!' It sounds simple, but positive self-talk as a reward is so easily done, yet so easily missed! Another form of reward is sharing your success and progress with a loved one who you know will respond positively.

While your rewards don't need to be physical, some of you might prefer this. For example, if you sustain a new behaviour for a whole week, buy or do something that you really like, such as getting a massage, buying a lippy or nail polish, or treating yourself to a new book or journal. Whatever small or large thing that motivates you will suffice.

4. Routines

Doing your new behaviour at a set time every day is helpful for habit formation, which is more powerful than willpower and motivation alone. So, experiment. See if you can find some way to build a regular routine or ritual around your new behaviour so it starts to become part of your way of life. For example, if you drive home from work, then every night, just before you get out of your car, you might do two minutes of mindful breathing and reflect on what values you want to live by when you walk through the front door into your home.

Take a look at my advice on completing the stress cycle in the next section (*see* p. 194) – completing the stress cycle is a ritualised act that you do to separate your work day from your home life, and it is a great way to start to build a new, helpful but achievable routine.

5. Relationships

I've already outlined the importance of good relationships for successful burnout recovery. Having someone to support you will make behaviour change easier. On the flip side, if the people around you are unsupportive, it will make it very hard.

Challenge yourself to find a kind, caring, encouraging person who can support you with your new behaviour and help you to be accountable. Maybe you can check in with this person on a regular basis and tell them how well you are doing. When I was trying to engage in changes after burnout, I would ask my husband to help keep me on track and gently point out when I was falling into old, unhelpful patterns of thinking and behaviour. It really helped.

6. Reflecting

Regularly take time to reflect on how you are behaving and what effect it is having on your life. You can do this by writing it down (records) or in discussion with another person (relationships). Or, carry it out as a mental exercise, either throughout the day, just before you go to bed or as you wake up in the morning.

Simply take a few moments to reflect on questions such as:

- How am I behaving?
- What am I doing that's working
- What am I doing that's not working?
- What can I do more of, less of, or differently?

Make sure you also reflect on the times that you stop doing the new behaviour and fall back into the old one. Notice what triggers those relapses and setbacks, and non-judgementally reflect on the genuine costs to your health and well-being caused by falling back into old habits. This will motivate you to get back on track.

7. Restructuring

This can sometimes be difficult to do in workplaces that cause burnout, but restructuring environments will make behaviour changes easier to sustain.

To give an example, if your new behaviour is going to the gym every morning before work, put your gym clothes out the night before so that you can get dressed easily first thing and place your kit bag and work stuff by the front door. In doing this you're removing structural problems (albeit relatively small ones) that might stop you from practising the new habit.

Admittedly, this is harder to do in burnout and at work, so your environment restructuring might involve changing when, where or how you interact with people that you know will push your boundaries and have negative effects on your behaviour change.

Exercise 46

Just one change
Pick one change that is important for to you to prioritise after burnout. Which of the seven Rs are you going to use to help you sustain this change?

Bonus Step 1: Staying Healthy After Change

I have supported many people through burnout. I know where they typically get stuck in their recoveries and I will give a range of strategies here for overcoming the most common problems. Pick and choose what you need from the following advice:

- How to maintain your recovery through utilising your rest time and hobbies effectively after burnout, covering:
  - Breaks during the work day
  - Breaks outside of work
  - Completing the stress cycle
  - How to use your hobbies to maintain recovery
- How to maintain your recovery by managing your stress levels after burnout, covering:
  - Three ways to monitor your stress levels after burnout
  - Three techniques to manage acute stress successfully
  - Writing a mental health toolkit to help you manage ongoing stress
  - What to do if you think you're sliding back into burnout.

These additional changes are complementary to the hard work you will already have done in addressing your workplace and individual factors after burnout. They will work nicely alongside any techniques you have learned in therapy, too. Think of them as the cherry on top of your recovery cake – you've already done the hard work creating a good foundation for maintaining your recovery; these are the finishing touches!

How to Maintain Your Recovery Through Utilising Your Rest Time and Hobbies Effectively after Burnout

Burnout fundamentally changes your stamina and ability to cope with stress at work. After burnout, you'll most likely be more fatigued after work and will need longer to recover between shifts. I can't tell you how important it is to factor adequate rest and recovery time both into your work day and life outside of work. It's a fundamental part of the early days of your recovery journey, and if you get it wrong you will struggle with absolutely everything else that follows.

Breaks During the Work Day

Once you've made changes to how you work, you need to pay attention to how you take your rest and downtime. Think about how you can structure your work to allow for this. In what ways are you going to change how you take rest during the working day and between your shifts?

Overwhelmingly, research suggests that frequent daily recovery efforts are more important and effective than waiting for the weekend or a less-frequent but longer annual holiday. Hands up if you've been on holiday and felt amazing while you were away, then when you come back to work, within a few short hours of being back, you're feeling as stressed as you were before! While holidays might help you feel temporarily better, their effects are not maintained on return.

Regular short breaks during the working day are also better in burnout recovery than taking a single long lunch break.

How you achieve this will entirely be down to how much flexibility you have over your work schedule, and some of you will have more control over this than others. If you're able to do so, the Pomodoro® Technique is a fabulous way of ensuring that you have frequent breaks, whilst maximising productivity. With this technique, you select a single task to work on, set a timer for 25–30 minutes, and work continuously until the timer goes off. You then get up, get a drink/go for a walk/have a stretch for 5 minutes, and then return to your tasks. Repeat for 4 rounds then take a longer 20–30-minute break. If the Pomodoro® Technique is not suitable for your work environment (unfortunately, this technique doesn't work in all settings), I suggest aiming for a short 5–10-minute break every couple of hours, and a longer break every 4–6 hours, if possible.

Breaks Outside of Work

So many people with burnout find it hard to accept that rest needs to happen, and crucially, rest needs to be just that – rest. I definitely got caught up in my own expectation that rest should be as 'productive' and driven as my time at work, and I've had to do an awful lot to undo that pattern of thinking and accept that not only is rest and proper downtime good, it's essential.

Your rest time at home's really important to get right. In today's modern era, where we have access to smartphones and emails, we are far too easily contactable. Our home lives are often interrupted by our work lives. In burnout it's smartphone use, in particular, that will hamper your recovery. Specifically, receiving text messages or WhatsApp notifications about work and actively checking emails after work hours. Sometimes we check our emails without even realising what we're doing until it's too late, just because we're in that habit. Thinking about work reduces your ability to recover from it, so the argument is that even the *presence* of a mobile phone can be a distraction!

The key here is to detach yourself mentally and physically from work after your workday has ended. Close your laptop and walk away, then put your phone in another room when you get home. This is quite difficult for people who work from home to achieve, so if you work from home, have a separate space – if you can – away from the normal living arrangements from where you work. That way, when work is done, you can walk away, shut the door, close your laptop (whatever it is symbolically that you do to remove yourself from your work in the home) and start to rest.

Completing the Stress Cycle

One of my favourite techniques to help separate work and home life is to do an exercise called completing the stress cycle, which was first described in the book, *Burnout* by Amelia and Emily Nagoski.

Completing the stress cycle is a ritualised act that you do every time you finish work. Once you start doing it regularly, your body will learn to recognise that particular act as a signal to your body, that your work day is over, your stress is over and you can start to relax. There are lots of different ways that you can do this – some of which will be more accessible than others – but there really is something for everyone.

I like to do some movement if I can, so I'll either go for a walk or to an exercise class. This is not always possible, owing to my schedule and family commitments, but that's how I like to do it. Sometimes I like to paint my nails because obviously, being a clinician, it's not advised from an infection control point of view, so, for me, it's a little act of rebellion. When I put nail polish on, I know that I'm not going to be working and that's a huge mindset shift for me.

Exercise 47

 How can you complete the stress cycle?
Think about what act you can do every time you finish work to help with completing the stress cycle.

Some people might get changed, have a shower or enjoy a herbal tea when they come in from work. Others might like to put on a loud piece of music and dance. If none of that feels appropriate or accessible to you, you can choose to sit or lie quietly, clench all of your muscles as hard and as tight as you can and hold, hold, hold... then relax. Do this again and again until you feel your mind begin to slow down and your body start to relax.

How to Use Your Hobbies to Maintain Recovery

In burnout, learning or mastering a new skill outside of work can help with recovery and will also improve your performance at work. It might feel counterintuitive that further drawing on your depleted energy and resources during non-work periods will benefit your recovery, but we know that mastering skills outside of work, such as learning a new language or playing a musical instrument, helps you generate new skills and replenishes depleted resources that can then be applied back into your work life.

When you start thinking about the sort of skills you'd like to learn, it's important that you don't fall into the trap of doing something that is linked to your work. Things like doing an extra project or audit, learning leadership skills or going on a course, for example, are too close to your work to be beneficial for recovery. For learning a new skill to truly have a benefit in burnout recovery, it needs to be completely uncoupled from work. You also need to be fairly established in your recovery process, because if you do it early on in your burnout, you're not going to have the energy or capacity to do it. Mastering a new skill requires high levels of dedication, focus and time.

Creativity is important in encouraging flow state, when you're so engrossed in a task that you lose sense of time passing by. I'm sure that you will all identify with having done an activity where you suddenly look up at the clock and realise that hours have passed, when it felt like minutes. This is a form of mindfulness by itself, which can be really helpful for burnout recovery.

What skill could you learn outside of work? (If you can make it creative at the same time, all the better.) You could join a choir, take up painting or pottery, or learn a new sport or outdoor pursuit. I learned to sew and make my own clothes – not only has this helped my burnout recovery, I now also have a fabulous post-burnout wardrobe that is entirely made to measure. (I also happen to have a heap of failed projects, but every single one of them has been a valuable learning exercise!) I find getting into the flow state quite easy with sewing and it really helps to focus and quieten my mind.

Exercise 48

 Put hobbies into play
Think about what new skill or creative pursuit you are interested in learning. What first steps do you need to take to make this a reality?

How to Maintain Your Recovery by Managing Your Stress Levels after Burnout

It might sound simple to talk about the early warning signs of stress overload, but if you've burned out previously then you will have missed those warning signs before and will be all too aware that it is much easier to recognise them in hindsight. One of the key changes you will need to make after burnout is not just how you handle your stress, but how often you monitor your stress levels.

Three Ways to Monitor Your Stress Levels after Burnout

You must develop a way of regularly monitoring your stress levels after burnout. How you chose to do this is entirely up to you – you might like to journal, you might like to use your smart watch to digitally track parameters such as heart rate variability – whatever it is, you need to be able to use it regularly. When you do this regularly, coupled with an awareness of your early warning signs of stress overload, you'll have a robust way of monitoring your stress levels after burnout, *and* know when to take action.

My early warning signs of increasing stress are:

- Nightmares (this is normally the first sign)
- Grinding my teeth overnight
- Finding it hard to get off to sleep because my mind is racing
- Fatigue (regardless of the quantity or quality of sleep)
- Tension headaches
- Irritability and pessimism
- Catastrophising
- Procrastinating

If I'm feeling under pressure but I don't have any of the above symptoms, then I know that I'm handling my stress well. However, if I'm under pressure and I develop any of the above symptoms, this is a trigger for me to think about how I am handling my stress. I'll take action to either improve how I'm coping (for example, by trying different therapeutic techniques) or to make practical changes to reduce my stress levels (for example, by seeing if I can change my present workload). It's important that you have this awareness too.

Exercise 49

Know the signs of stress
Write down:

- the physical symptoms you get when you are increasingly stressed;
- the thoughts you have when you are increasingly stressed;
- how your behaviour changes when you're stressed. For example, do you exercise less or drink more alcohol? Or perhaps you end up withdrawing from seeing friends and family or working longer hours. Referring back to your early burnout symptoms (*see* p. 22) might help you here.

Now you have an idea about how the symptoms of stress overload present in yourself, you need to find a way of consciously monitoring how you are feeling on a regular basis. Here are three ways that you could do this:

1. Regular Journaling

Not only is journaling a fantastic way of monitoring your stress levels after burnout but it can also be a helpful technique for managing your anxiety and depression and reducing stress. Interestingly, time spent journaling about our deepest thoughts and feelings can even reduce the number of sick days we take off work.

Writing things down:

- helps to prioritise problems, fears and concerns;
- allows you to monitor any day-to-day symptoms;
- keeps a track of symptoms, so you can recognise triggers and learn better ways to manage them;
- provides an opportunity for positive self-talk;
- identifies negative thoughts and behaviour;
- helps us to accept rather than judge our mental experiences, resulting in fewer negative emotions in response to stresses.

So, it's a great habit to get into after burnout.

If you would like to journal, then how regularly you chose to write is entirely up to you. The more frequently you do it, the bigger the benefits. When I'm stressed I tend to journal daily or every other day, and when I'm well I do less of it. You only need to carve out five to ten minutes a day to feel the benefits.

2. Burnout Questionnaires

Rather than journaling, some of you may prefer to do validated questionnaires to monitor your stress levels. You could choose to regularly review the five stages of burnout (*see* p. 96) and see if you identify with any of them. You can also regularly redo burnout questionnaires to help you monitor for any sign of change.

However, as change is slow in burnout recovery, don't get hung up on any results or numbers or be disheartened if your scores aren't shifting. I'd recommend waiting two to three months between repeating your burnout scores. How you feel in yourself and learning to be in tune with your emotional state is arguably a better way to know if your recovery is moving in the right direction.

3. Wearables and Digital Stress Tracking

You can also monitor your stress levels using wearables and tracking via apps. The advantage to this approach is that there is less effort on your part to track – all you have to do is put your wearable on, and off you go! However, it's essential to know what you're going to do with the data you get from wearables, rather than monitoring just for the sake of it!

I would never recommend using one or two of these measures as the sole indicator of your stress levels, but they can be really helpful for alerting you that you might need to take action to bring your stress levels down. I use the free version of an app called Welltory, which I use with my Apple Watch, but there are lots of different apps and devices you can chose from.

Exercise 50

Monitor your stress levels

Pick a single technique to monitor your stress levels on a regular basis. Where, when and how frequently are you going to monitor them?

Three Techniques to Manage Acute Stress Successfully

There will be moments in your recovery when you feel the familiar sensations of your 'fight or flight' response rearing its ugly head once more. I vividly remember starting a shift over a bank holiday weekend at a busy urgent care centre. Looking at the screen and seeing the hundreds of patients that required call backs and appointments, my heart started racing and my palms began sweating. I felt physically sick and completely unable to start my work owing to internal panic.

In that moment, I took myself off to make a quick cup of tea. I stood in the kitchenette practising a defusion technique that I had learned during therapy (*see* p. 137). I took about five minutes, then – feeling calmer – I pulled myself together and got on with my work. And, do you know, the shift ended up being fine and the work was manageable. Overcoming that feeling of overwhelm at work was a huge milestone for me. I was so proud of myself for being able to stop that spiral into panic. I would not have been able to do that in the burnout period or early on in recovery.

It's essential that you also have some techniques that you can pull out in the moment that you feel overwhelmed, too. Here is a selection of three of my personal favourites:

1. Box Breathing

This technique helps to slow your heart rate down and overcome the physical sensations of overwhelm in the moment that it affects you. It's so effective that the Navy Seals are taught it to use in service. I used this technique just before a scary and important clinical exam where I could feel my heart racing in my chest, and it was helpful.

* Breathe in slowly for four counts.
* Hold at the top for four counts.
* Breathe out slowly for four counts.
* Hold at the bottom for four counts.
* Repeat until you feel calmer.

2. Physiological sigh

Similar to box breathing, this technique helps to slow your heart rate down.

* Rapidly breathe in through the nose, then do a second breath (i.e. do a double inhale)
* Exhale loudly through the mouth
* Repeat until you feel calmer.

3. Dropping Anchor

This is an effective grounding technique to do in the moment when you feel overwhelmed with emotion. Refer back to Exercise 33 (p. 139) for instructions on how to do this.

Exercise 51

Act to prevent overwhelm

Think about what you can do in the moment when you start to feel panicky, stressed and overwhelmed at work. Which act or exercise helps you the most? Pick one to try the next time this happens to you.

Writing a Mental Health Toolkit to Help You Manage Ongoing Stress

It is important to know when you need to start doing deep work. The key here is about how much your mood is affecting your function, your relationships and your performance at work, how your quality of life is affected by your stress and how sustained it is. Hopefully you now have some of the tools to be able to recognise this. If your function or performance at work, quality of life or relationships are being consistently affected by a dip in mood or prolonged stress, then you need to seek professional help from your doctor or a psychologist. But, there will be a point prior to this where you can help yourself by using your mental health toolkit and the skills that you've already got.

A good mental health toolkit is one that contains things that you know help you when you're feeling low or stressed, and are specific, measurable and easily actionable. For instance, 'being kind to yourself' isn't a specific, measurable or easily actionable tool. However, 'listening to a self-compassion audio exercise' is, and this is far easier to implement and feel the benefits of. Do some reflective work now about what you know has helped you the most during your burnout, and then go back to those techniques when things feel difficult.

While compiling a toolkit might feel a little formal, knowing what to reach or who to turn to if you notice your stress levels are rising and you might be at risk of burnout again is important. Your toolkit can be physical, virtual or a combination of both. It will be completely unique to you and you need to work out what will help you to make you feel better when you're feeling low.

What Should Your Toolkit Include?

Ideally, you should have a combination of tools that cover all four of these categories:

1. **Physical health** – for example, exercise and movement, sleep and nutrition.
2. **Relationships** – for example, peer support, your loved ones and professional support.
3. **Mindset** – for example, practising therapy techniques, meditation, mindfulness, self-care and prayer.
4. **Preventing self-neglect** – for example, going to medical appointments and taking your medications.

Here are some physical items you might wish to include in your mental health toolkit:

- A journal
- A comforting book
- Numbers of people to call when you are struggling
- Photos of people and places you love and feel safe with
- Comfy clothes
- A warm weighted blanket
- Sleep aids
- White noise
- Mindful colouring books
- A knitting or crochet project
- Jigsaws

You could also include virtual items. Write down a reminder to:

- watch a familiar, much-loved TV programme;
- dance or play loud music;
- try therapy techniques that work for you;
- have a massage;
- cuddle a pet;
- visit a place that has happy memories for you.

Exercise 52

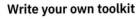

Write your own toolkit

Write down three things in each category (physical tools/relationship tools/mindset tools and prevention of self-neglect tools) that you know will help you to feel better when you're feeling low. Ensure that your relationship toolkit also contains the names of five people or communities that you can turn to for help in the moment. These might include the number of your doctor or a mental health helpline, for instance.

Whether your toolkit is physical or digital, keep it somewhere easily accessible.

What to Do if You Think You're Sliding Back into Burnout

Now you have an awareness of the signs of increasing stress in yourself and an idea about how to monitor your stress levels. You will also have picked some tools and techniques to help manage both acute and ongoing stress in order to maintain your recovery. Now let's move on to covering what you need to do if you think you're sliding back into burnout.

One of the hardest things I had to navigate during my recovery was the awful sense of dread I'd get whenever I felt stressed. I'd worry that the burnout was coming back whenever I had a difficult day at work. Knowing if (or when) you're starting to slide back into burnout is challenging, without doubt. Having days that are harder than others is part of navigating the spectrum that is normal mental health, even when you're not burned out, but after burnout the worry that you'll slide will likely be a constant concern.

Recovery is never linear or straightforward. The key thing is that you are able to recognise when a difficult or challenging day is not a temporary blip but a persistent change. If you've burned out before, you'll now know that you missed vital warning signs of worsening stress levels the first time around – I know I certainly did! Teacher Kirsty Sinclair reflects on her own experience of recovery:

Take time to decide what recovery means for you, and be ready to revise your opinion regularly. This will be regardless of what your friends or family might be expecting. Burnout has a metamorphic effect that forces sizeable decisions and changes, as well as revision of values. To attempt to return to what you were doing before, in the same way, is to invite a repeat experience. I found recovery wasn't a linear process. The outcome may bring the unexpected, but will undoubtedly broaden your horizons and accelerate personal growth. If you have dependents, whatever is best for you will probably ultimately be best for them too. Self-sacrifice is unsustainable.

The post-burnout period has to be one of change, paradoxically at a time when your reserves and capacity to make those changes is reduced. If you find that things are not working out, go back and work out which stage of recovery you are in again and restart the process from there. If you slide again it's a trigger for you to re-evaluate which changes were not sufficient previously. It's a painful and frustrating thing to experience, but this is what needs to be done. Sustaining that recovery you've worked *so* hard for doesn't mean a yoga class once a week; it means keeping up with the significant changes you've made and ensuring you're reviewing their effectiveness regularly.

It's fine to have the occasional difficult day, but if they start to become more persistent or consistent, or if you are starting to feel worse over time, you must take action. Please seek help from a doctor and/or therapist if you have a second (or multiple) burnouts.

Exercise 53

Identify and act if you're burning out again

Go back to p. 96, recap the five stages of burnout and do the Burnout Assessment Tool. What do your results tell you? If you are burning out again, can you identify the cause?

Was there anything that you missed in your recovery process (refer back to pp. 111–115 to help you identify what might have been overlooked).

What are the first steps that you need to take now to make things better?

Bonus Step 2: Identifying and Overcoming Barriers to Change

On your recovery journey, you are extremely likely to encounter resistance to change, both internally from within yourself and externally from the people and systems with which you work. It's the same as pretty much anything else that requires behavioural change... it doesn't matter if you're trying to quit smoking, prioritise sleep, lose weight, exercise more or recover from burnout, you *will* come up against powerful barriers to change. When you do, you're unfortunately much more likely to fall off the bandwagon. You cannot rely on your intrinsic sense of motivation alone to get better. In burnout, your motivation will already be depleted, and it's already very hard work to make the changes needed after burnout to help in recovery.

Early identification of any barriers to change will allow you to be far more effective with any changes you make. Anticipating these barriers in advance will help you to mitigate them and improve your chances of a successful recovery. Ideally, these powerful barriers to change must be worked through prior to going through with changes.

In this second bonus step, we're going to cover the things that will stop you recovering in two halves. The first half focuses on your internal barriers, such as cognitive biases, guilt and shame. The second half focuses on external and structural barriers, such as personal and professional relationships and your finances. Finally, we'll discuss how to effectively make difficult decisions about your future after burnout. Each factor discussed has practical tips and exercises to help you overcome whichever barriers you are currently facing. Pick out the strategies that are most relevant to you and your personal circumstances.

Internal Barriers to Recovery

Cognitive Biases

Cognitive biases are the ways that you think and the patterns of thinking that you inadvertently fall into that will hold you back from effective decision-making and change. Cognitive biases featured highly in my post-burnout decision-making and, without doubt, slowed my recovery down.

A cognitive bias is a systemic error that occurs in thinking when people are processing and interpreting information about the world around them, and it directly affects the decisions and judgements that they make. The brain is incredibly powerful, but it is subject to limitations. A cognitive bias is a strong preconceived notion of something or someone based on information that we have perceived to have or are missing. But these preconceptions are essentially mental shortcuts that the brain takes in order to speed up and improve information processing. The aim is to help the brain quickly make sense of what it is seeing and sensing.

These errors in how we think may not always be done intentionally or consciously. This then makes it difficult for us to process accurate information and to work out the truth. It distorts our critical thinking, and it possibly leads to perpetuating misconceptions or misinformation. It might lead us to avoid information that might be unwelcome or uncomfortable, rather than investigating information that might lead us to a more accurate outcome. It also causes us to see patterns or connections between ideas that aren't necessarily there.

Cognitive biases are really powerful, even for people that haven't burned out. In burnout, your brain function and structure has already been altered, albeit temporarily, and therefore your patterns of thinking have changed already, meaning that it will be even trickier to avoid some of these biases.

There are many studied and named cognitive biases, but there are some which feature more predominately in burnout, which are helpful for you to know. These are the sunk cost fallacy, commitment bias, choice overload and status quo bias.

The Sunk Cost Fallacy

Have you ever been told in a moment of indecision about your career, 'You can't give up now, you've put so much time and effort into this'? Well, this happens to be the sunk cost fallacy in action!

The sunk cost fallacy describes the tendency to follow through on a decision if we have already invested time, effort or money into it, regardless of whether or not the current costs outweigh the benefits. This is true of any career where you have invested time, energy, emotions and finances into training. In my case this was medicine, but there are many other careers or vocations that require high levels of investment, such as law, teaching and nursing.

The sunk cost fallacy means that you fall into a particularly vicious cycle where you *continue* to invest time, money and effort into the decisions and choices that you've already invested in, even if that particular decision is *not* the right thing for you to continue to do. The more that's invested, the more you feel committed to continuing that pursuit and the greater resources you are likely to put in to follow through on your decision, even if it's not the right choice for you anymore. In burnout, the sunk cost fallacy potentially prevents us from making the right career choices and decisions that are essential for recovery; particularly so if you are a high-achieving professional and have invested a lot into getting to your current position.

Focusing on past investments instead of the present and future costs and benefits means that you end up committing to decisions that are no longer in your best interests or serve you after burnout. Part of the reason why people get so sucked into the sunk cost fallacy is because of loss aversion, which describes the fact that the impact of losses feels much stronger to us than the impact of gains. Therefore, we are more likely to avoid losses than seek out gains. If you feel that your past investment will be lost if you don't follow through on your original decision or commitment, you're much more likely to make a decision based on loss aversion. In this case, it's better to consider the benefits that would be gained if you do not continue your commitment.

In burnout, it is helpful to remember that your investment has got you into a position of harm, and that any next steps you take will be made *because* of your investment, not in spite of it. It's helpful to bear this in mind if your family is also invested in your career, whether this is financially, emotionally or both.

How to Manage the Sunk Cost Fallacy

If you are aware that you are continuing to make a decision because of previous past investments, shift from focusing on what you've done in the past to the *current costs and benefits* of making a decision. Don't look at what you've already done; concentrate on the here and now, and any potential future gains.

Focus on taking concrete actions and writing a roadmap, rather than on the feeling of wastefulness or guilt that accompanies dropping an earlier commitment. This will help to remove some of the emotion from uncoupling yourself from your past investments in burnout, particularly if you have a vocational career.

Be prepared for push back from loved ones, especially if you come from a background where you were pushed to achieve academically and went into a career where you were trying to please your parents instead of yourself. Practise any difficult conversations in advance (*see* p. 185 for more on this) so that you feel ready and strong.

Commitment Bias

Similar to the sunk cost fallacy, commitment bias describes our tendency to remain committed to our past behaviours and choices, particularly if they have been exhibited publicly. In this bias, commitment continues to be shown to the original decision, even if the outcome of the decision has not been demonstrated to be desirable. You continue to stand by that choice because it has been publicly exhibited and (rather understandably) you don't want to lose face. This is slightly different to the sunk cost fallacy, where you are continuing to be committed to something because of the *investment* that you've put into it.

Commitment bias is perpetuated a lot in vocational careers, and it generally prevents us from making good decisions post-burnout. To give an example, when doctors get into medical school, they tend to tell as many friends and family as they can about it. If they then go on to burn out, commitment bias is something that might stop them from changing their chosen career path (if this is what they need or want) because they've so publicly exhibited commitment previously. The commitment bias really comes into play if you are considering whether or not to leave your job.

How to Manage Commitment Bias

A lot of tackling commitment bias is about giving yourself permission to make significant changes free from guilt (more about guilt later, *see* p. 214). So, if you find that certain past publicly exhibited behaviours or commitments of yours no longer align with your current post-burnout values or goals, there is absolutely no reason to stick with them. We are allowed to grow and change as humans. It's natural to worry that others will think less of us if our decisions lead to negative outcomes or are inconsistent with our previous decision-making. But, in fact, people actually have more respect for those that are able to admit that something's gone wrong. There will always be people that disagree with you, of course, and sometimes they might be very close to you. Managing the disappointment of others is difficult, but ultimately the decision to change really doesn't affect anyone but yourself.

If this is difficult (and I know it will be for many of you, particularly if you have families that will be disappointed if you want to change career path), I recommend having some CBT or ACT to help you find some coping strategies (*see* p. 136).

Choice Overload

Choice overload is also known as the paradox of choice, and it describes how people become overwhelmed when they are presented with a large number of options to choose from. We live in a hyper-consumerist, instant-gratification society, and often the assumption is that choice makes us happy. In fact, the opposite happens when you have lots of choice. Our brains are unable to cope and we get overwhelmed.

In burnout you will already be feeling overwhelmed. One of the key parts of burnout recovery – once you have sufficiently restored your health – is exploring your work options. In this stage of recovery most people explore multiple options, but the danger here is falling into choice overload.

Choice overload makes it harder to make effective decisions. You can feel so overwhelmed that you end up putting off the decision and just giving up or indefinitely procrastinating.

In burnout, you have to make change. You have to make difficult choices. You have to follow through on those decisions if you want to sustain your recovery. Having lots of choices isn't necessarily bad in itself, rather it becomes harmful when you are simultaneously trying to learn about all of your options and make a decision about them at the same time.

How to Manage Choice Overload

Give yourself permission to browse without the intention of committing. When people go into shops with the intention of browsing – without putting any pressure on themselves to commit to one option – they are less likely to end up feeling the effects of cognitive overload. When you're thinking about your post-burnout career, give yourself permission to just have a look at all of the options. You don't have to make a decision straight away, and it's better to just relieve yourself of that immediate pressure.

When it does come to making a decision, the best way to manage choice overload is to try to avoid regret by treating your choices as non-reversible, even if they technically aren't. Very few decisions are non-reversible – and certainly in burnout, quite a lot of our options available to us don't have to be permanent – but it's best treated as though they are. This will help avoid buyer's remorse.

Keep a gratitude journal and focus on the positives of the decision you've made.

Status Quo Bias

Status quo bias refers to our innate preference as human beings for the current state of affairs – even if the current state of affairs is harming us – resulting in resistance to change. Everyone knows the saying, 'If it ain't broke, don't fix it' – this is the status quo bias! But, in burnout, things really *are* broken and you *do* need to fix them. Even if staying where you are feels safe and familiar, you have to make change.

In burnout, the status quo bias might lead you to avoid making a decision or simply opt for the default option because you're feeling overwhelmed by the number or complexity of options available to you. Opting towards the status quo helps you to avoid the stress of making a decision (and, in burnout, you're already stressed with limited energy and capacity for decision-making).

How to Manage Status Quo Bias

You can actively avoid falling into the suboptimal default by making a plan of action and writing a roadmap. Setting some effective SMARTR goals (*see* p. 174) or writing a career development plan (*see* p. 161) will help in this case.

Exercise 54

Cognitive biases and you

Think about which bias(es) have the most impact on your decision-making at this time. What one thing can you start today to make a difference to their impact on your decision-making?

Mindset

The other thing that can hold you back from good decisions post-burnout is your mindset. The first book that I read after my burnout (well, I say read, but I dipped in and out because I had very little energy or concentration) was *Mindset* by the psychologist, Carol Dweck. This book honestly changed my outlook and how I felt about my decision-making moving forward in my burnout.

In a fixed mindset, you believe that your intelligence and talents are fixed and static. Conversely, in a growth mindset, you believe that your intelligence and talents can be improved through effort and learning. In a fixed mindset if you're not good at something you'll likely believe that you'll never be good at it, whereas the opposite happens in a growth mindset. This matters in burnout because the consequences of thinking that your intelligence or personality is something that is a fixed, deep-seated trait – versus thinking that it can grow and be developed – will deeply affect your outlook and decision-making skills. If you believe your qualities are unchangeable, you'll want to prove yourself and will fall into correcting yourself over and over, rather than really learning from your mistakes.

A person with a fixed mindset usually avoids challenges in life. They give up easily and become intimidated or threatened by the success of others. This is in part because in a fixed mindset you believe that intelligence and talent is not something that you can develop; it's something that you *are*, that you're born with and that you cannot change. This leads to negative thinking.

In burnout, when you start to find things hard at work, you will very likely start to berate yourself about this. You might blame yourself and say to yourself, 'It's my fault', 'I'm not smart enough', 'Why can't I just cope?' This was exactly how I spoke in my head to myself during burnout – there was so much negative self-talk. Where, previously, I very much had a growth mindset, I fell into a fixed mindset as a result of my burnout process.

Changing my mindset helped me to move away from a fear of failure and fruitlessly trying to correct the mistakes that I'd made in my burnout, to work harder and to stay in the same job. There was a lot of guilt and a lot of shame. Because I had a fixed mindset, I genuinely thought that my burnout had happened because of some inherent fault in me. I was so ashamed, I wasn't in a position to try to grow and learn from my mistakes. Switching to a growth mindset opened up so many opportunities for me. Changing your beliefs has such a powerful impact post-burnout. Why waste time trying to prove to yourself over and over that you are worthy when you could be putting what precious little energy you have into getting better?

A growth mindset views intelligence and talent as qualities that can be developed. This doesn't mean that people with a growth mindset assume they're going to be the next Einstein; there are still variables in what we can all achieve. A growth mindset simply means that people believe that their intelligence and talent can be improved through effort and action. It recognises that setbacks are a necessary part of the learning process and it allows people to bounce back by increasing motivational effort. This mindset sees failings as temporary and changeable.

A growth mindset is crucial for learning resilience, motivation, performance and burnout recovery. And if you adapt to the growth mindset, you are more likely to embrace lifelong learning, put in more effort to learn, and believe the effort leads to mastery. With a growth mindset, you will believe that failures are just temporary setbacks. You will willingly embrace challenges, view other successes as a source of inspiration and treat feedback as an opportunity to learn. A growth mindset doesn't just help with recovery in burnout, it also helps improve motivation and academic performance, and reduces depression and anxiety.

How to move towards a growth mindset

The first thing I would recommend is reading Carol Dweck's *Mindset*. It's really liberating in burnout to move from thinking that you are a failure to realising that your mistakes are part of a learning journey and are an opportunity for you to grow and create a better life, a better career. Learn to believe the good things that you are told using the CBT thought diary.

Exercise 55

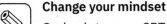

Change your mindset

Go back to your CBT diary (as outlined on p. 135). Whenever you experience any negative associated thoughts in burnout, capture it then write it down. Then, write a new alternative thought for you to believe in. If you want to go one step further, you could write a new compelling belief in your own skills, attributes and capacity for positive change.

Unhelpful Thinking Styles

Please refer to p. 131 for more information on unhelpful thinking styles, and how to successfully overcome them.

Guilt and Shame

Guilt and shame directly impact on both burnout development and recovery. I know this because I've been there and experienced it myself, but also because on social media and in my discussions with other people with burnout this is a topic that comes up repeatedly. It's an issue that particularly affects those in caring professions or positions that carry significant responsibility, but, crucially, it can also affect others.

Guilt

Guilt is implicated in both the development of burnout and in negatively impacting recovery. In fact, the experience of guilt is linked so closely to burnout that it has been speculated that it should be added to its symptoms and definition in order to distinguish between burnout and alternative mental health diagnoses.

Before you can look to overcome guilt in burnout, it's essential that you have an understanding about how guilt can work against you. Guilt is the feeling of having committed a wrongdoing or failed in an obligation, or a sense of responsibility or remorse for an event, whether real or imagined. In some ways, guilt has advantages for professionals – in particular those in caring or health professions or positions of responsibility – as it promotes empathy, meticulousness and hard work. However, it can also unfortunately lead to negative thoughts or behaviours, such as exerting undue pressure on ourselves, being excessively critical and worrying often. This is something that gets wildly out of control in burnout. Furthermore, the guilt experienced will almost certainly not be caused by any wrongdoing. The guilt in burnout is therefore *inappropriate* for the situation.

The guilt you feel so strongly and urgently in burnout is overwhelmingly unlikely to be appropriate guilt, i.e., you experience it *because of the burnout process* not because you've done anything wrong. When you experience this inappropriate guilt, you won't necessarily make the conscious link to it being inappropriate to anything you may or may not have done. The way you feel because of this inappropriate guilt is the same as when the guilt is appropriate, and it therefore drives you to patterns of thinking and behaviours that look on the surface to be helpful but in fact are worsening your burnout or hampering your recovery.

For instance, if you are stressed at work but not yet burned out, you might find yourself working longer hours and feeling that you can't say no to additional work because you feel this guilt. Remember Stage 2 of burnout (*see* p. 97) and the three hallmark features of this stage: seeing friends and family less, feeling that your work is the most important thing in your life, and lack of time for personal needs. Inappropriate guilt will likely be factoring into these thoughts and behavioural changes, which in turn hastens the speed of the decline into Stages 4 and 5.

For those that are in burnout, or habitual burnout, the experience of inappropriate guilt might stop you from making helpful decisions about your recovery, such as taking time off sick or reaching out for help. This is definitely something that I experienced myself; I couldn't bring myself to take sick leave when I first burned out, even though I desperately needed to. Guilt about the impact my absence would have on my patients and colleagues was a huge factor in my decision-making. I didn't realise that the guilt wasn't because of any poor patient care or negligence, but through persistent self-tortures, the burnout process itself as well as organisational pressures.

The experience of inappropriate guilt in burnout can also be a huge problem even if you don't work in a vocational or caring job. Dan Bartlett, former tech co-founder and Head of Engineering, describes his own experience of guilt in burnout:

I would think things like: other people have children and busy jobs and they're doing fine; only carers, doctors and nurses get real burnout; I'm

just sat on a laptop all day, and I'm paid well for it. These thoughts left
me feeling confused and helpless, because regardless of what 'should'
have been happening, I was in so much pain. This was compounded at
[the second job after burnout] because the work/life balance was much
better than my last job. So I blamed myself for how hard everything felt.
I felt unworthy of feeling unworthy.

What helped? Trusting my intuition that something wasn't right,
alongside research that helped me understand how long it can take
to recover from burnout, how bad it can get, and that burnout doesn't
discriminate

Guilt is, as you can see, an integral part of the burnout experience, regardless of the profession that you work in. It doesn't matter where you work or what job you do. It doesn't matter if you're better paid than other people or if your job doesn't involve so-called 'worthy' work. The experience is the same, as it's the end point of prolonged stress.

This inappropriately experienced guilt will impact directly on every single stage of your recovery journey, *unless* you take action to address it. Guilt about any impact on your colleagues or others that might be affected by your absence might stop you from taking time off work when you desperately need to. If you do go off sick, guilt might drive you back to work before you're ready. Guilt will also stop you from resting appropriately during the restoration of health stage of recovery. It will prevent you from working out your true values, exploring the career options you want to, and making and maintaining significant changes at work.

Kirsty Sinclair explains how guilt affected her:

I had several false starts that created unsettling peaks and troughs.
I put great pressure on myself to recover quickly, as I panicked about
survival, money, what people would think of me and my sense of
vulnerability. The emotions were very difficult, there was a great deal

of guilt, shame and shock. What I didn't have for a long time was self-compassion and the depth of self-knowledge that I have now.

Shame

Guilt is linked to shame, and the experience of shame and vulnerability also directly impacts on our working lives (particularly in caring professions). For people that burn out, often their work forms a crucial part of their identity, and this strong attachment means it can be very difficult to separate shameful experiences from the self.

Shame is an intense, powerful emotion that taps into our deep-rooted fears that we're not good enough as people and that we're not good enough for our work. Shame prevents us from fully connecting with others, from living the life we want to lead and working in the way are capable of. Again, it's not just something that is experienced internally in burnout, it can also be externally applied. Open judgement and shaming still happens in the workplace whether people are in mental difficulty or struggling with burnout.

My own experience of shame prevented me from reaching out to my doctor during my burnout. The thought of explaining to them that I couldn't do the same job that they themselves were doing – the shame was just too much to bear. The surgery I am registered to is absolutely wonderful and the staff are caring and compassionate, so I would like to make it clear that this shame was 100 per cent in my head and not due to any negative experience. I was able to overcome this shame and get the medical help I needed by going through a different organisation that is commissioned to provide medical help and therapy for doctors. There, I felt relatively anonymous and could cope a little easier with the guilt and the shame, although it still affected me deeply. Subsequently, going through therapy helped me to address the guilt and shame I was experiencing, and I would highly recommend that you do the same if this is accessible to you.

The following exercises will help get you started in successfully tackling guilt, regardless of which stage of burnout or burnout recovery you are in.

Exercise 56

Experiencing guilt – journal prompts
Think about the following:

- Which specific situations at work cause you pain?
- What is the purpose of the guilt you're feeling? Is this justified?
- How is the guilt you're experiencing influencing your behaviours in unhelpful ways?
- What steps can you take to start to change the behaviours that are directly influenced by your experience of guilt?

Write down one action you can take this week to combat your feelings of guilt.

Exercise 57

Rephrase your inner criticisms
Rephrasing negative self-talk is a powerful weapon against guilt becoming a shaming experience.

When you get a thought of guilt, for example: 'I feel that I am a terrible person because I don't have the capacity to take on an extra shift', rephrase it to yourself into to a more positive and compassionate statement, for example: 'It is essential that I am rested physically and mentally in order to show up and be my best self at work.'

Exercise 58

Treat yourself as you would a good friend
Think about a time when a close friend felt really bad about themselves and came to you for help. How did you respond? Write down what you did, what you said and the way that it was delivered.

Now think about times when you feel bad about yourself or are struggling. How do you typically respond to yourself in these situations? Write down what you do, what you say and how it is delivered.

What are the differences between how you might help a friend that is struggling vs how you help yourself? What factors or fears come into play that lead you to treat yourself and others so differently?

Write down how you think things might change if you speak to yourself when you're suffering in the same way that you typically respond to a close friend.

Confidence

Burnout absolutely wrecks your confidence. At the height of my burnout, I constantly ruminated on decisions I was making about my patients because I had totally lost confidence in my abilities as a doctor, even though I was objectively performing fine at the time. I couldn't even get into the car to drive – a skill I'd had the entirety of my adult life – without being reduced to tears; such was my anxiety and lack of confidence.

Burnout really is a confidence killer. Even the most confident and assured people pre-burnout will experience this in burnout. And it matters when it comes to recovery because that loss of confidence might hold you back from making successful changes and advocating for yourself.

It took a long time for my confidence to come back. In fact, it was only in the latter stages of recovery – Phase Three, four years after my initial burnout – that I can say that it had returned. Your confidence will be something that returns late in this journey, and you cannot rush it. If you're much earlier in the burnout process, please put the precious limited energy you have into the things that are most important right now (such as rest, socialising, working on your values or exploring work options, depending on where you are in your recovery). The time to work on your confidence *will* come and you will get there. Have patience until you know you have the energy to do this.

Until you can work on genuinely *feeling* confident after burnout, start with improving confidence with your *actions* and *behaviour.* Admittedly, this is quite a scary thing to do, especially if your confidence is at rock bottom. To feel the fear, and go ahead with doing the thing you're not confident to do regardless, that's tough! However, I have wholeheartedly embraced this strategy, and let me tell you it's not easy but it definitely helps, especially when you start small and build up the fear factor over time.

Exercise 59

Step out of your comfort zone
Write some SMARTR goals (*see* p. 174), ensuring they are in alignment with your values (*see* p. 144). Pick one small action you can take today that pushes you slightly out of your comfort zone. Do it, then reflect on how you feel. Rinse and repeat, and over time this will help rebuild your confidence after burnout.

To change your thoughts of low confidence, I recommend starting with Exercise 31 (*see* p. 136). CBT-based exercises are great at getting you to consciously notice the critical thoughts that will be sapping your confidence and then to reframe them. Alternatively, you might choose to avoid challenging your thoughts, and instead you could do some ACT exercises to try to make space for them (*see* p. 137).

The following exercise also helps to identify your critical thoughts and work out what these help you to do and what they hold you back from.

Exercise 60

Catch your critic
Make a note of each time you experience a critical or confidence-lowering thought throughout the day in the table below. I've written an example for you:

Thought number	Time	Critical statement
1	8.30am	'I'm just not good enough.'

Review your thoughts at the end of the day and reflect on their purpose in this table:

Thought number	Helps me feel or do	Stops me feeling or doing
1	It did not help me to feel or do anything helpful.	Stops me feeling confident. Stops me doing what matters. Means I avoid putting myself forward for opportunities.

Then, reflect:

* Are there any recurring themes?
* Do these thoughts drive better performance or achievement?
* Do they discourage you from doing what you want to do?

Using this exercise, you should begin to understand when you are most critical, and subsequently start to challenge or reign in your inner critic.

External and Structural Barriers to Recovery: Your Support Networks

It's important that you are supported to recover from burnout and to both make and sustain the changes you need to be able to get better. If you don't get that support, it will be very difficult for you to achieve this.

The support I'm referring to is not only your immediate support networks (your immediate family, friends, peers and work colleagues) but also more formal structural and societal support (your GP, therapist, Employee Assistance Programme or occupational health department). Sadly, these support systems will not necessarily be accessible to everyone on an equal basis. The inequitable access to support might be based on your circumstances such as your socio-economic status, gender, ethnicity, sexuality or age. You support network might also include people that you employ to help ease the burden, such as a nanny or cleaner.

My bugbears with the advice typically given on social media on the topic of mental well-being are that it's often not accessible to all and it ignores the gaps in support that some people might face. A simple example of this might be a sleep-deprived working mum looking for advice on how to improve her sleep. The advice typically given focuses on what the evidence suggests she should do, such as go to bed at the same time each night; avoid screens, caffeine, alcohol and high-intensity exercise before bedtime; and sleep in a dark, cool and quiet room. This ignores the fact that she might be a single parent with two neurodiverse children who don't sleep through the night and she doesn't have local family to support her. For mums, often the advice is also fraught with judgement, which adds another layer of unnecessary complexity and guilt.

The same is true in burnout. You can plan all the changes in the world, but if you're not going to be supported and enabled to make those changes by the people around you – both at home and at work – you are not going to be successful. Your support network will make or break your recovery. Remember earlier in the book when I talked about the most significant predictors of burnout recovery, and good relationships was one of them (*see* p. 124)? When your support network is good and healthy, your burnout recovery will be that much easier; when your support network works against you, your recovery will be very difficult, if not impossible. So you have to consider your network. Are the people surrounding you helping or hindering your recovery?

Learning to Ask for Help

Learning to ask for help is tricky, but once you get going you'll be shocked at how easy it is. Hopefully you'll be pleasantly surprised by how much others will want to assist you. Often people simply don't know what they need to do, even if they want to help. If I know that someone is having difficulty, rather than saying something a bit vague but well-intentioned like, 'Let me know if there's anything I can help with', I'll ask specifically what will help them and see where that takes us in the conversation.

You need to identify what it is that you need help with and exactly what you need the people in your life to do. Think about what will have the most impact and go with that first. Ideally, start with something that doesn't require too much of others but will help you tremendously.

Proactive communication and being clear with your wants, needs and expectations is key, although this can be difficult in burnout when your confidence is shattered. Try to communicate what you need gently but assertively (more on empathetic assertiveness on p. 185) and be specific about the things you need, when you need them and how they need to be done.

Caring Responsibilities

While burnout is a workplace problem, I am a firm believer that it happens at the intersection of work stress with stressors and difficulties elsewhere in your life. Our capacity for stress is finite. We're a bit like sponges – we can absorb a lot of stress until we reach capacity and then the stress spills out uncontrollably.

Many of those who burn out will have additional caring responsibilities that then directly impact on their ability to make changes and recover. Caring for children or family members with additional needs, due to age, disability, emotional support or mental health problems are two situations that most obviously spring to mind. However, caring responsibilities can also take the form of financial support, such as sending money back to family abroad or supporting an adult child through university.

How do you successfully manage balancing the needs of your recovery with caring for others? A lot of our additional responsibilities – whether they are by choice or not – are things that we have to live with and work around, but these are not easily manageable or simple to tackle.

How to access support when you're a burned-out carer

Reach out for additional support from your network and ideally from people that get it themselves. The people who are in the same situation as you will understand it. Remember how peer support and community helps with burnout prevention and recovery (*see* pp. 49 and 124).

- If you're a single parent, can you talk to other single parents? What help do they get? Can you talk to your family? What help can they provide?

- If you're a carer, can you talk to other carers in the same situation as you?
- If you've got additional responsibilities, what help can you get? What can you afford to outsource?
- If you've got young children, what additional childcare can you access in order to help you recover?

If you can't outsource help to tackle your specific additional responsibility, are there other things you can outsource to ease the burden in other parts of your life and help you concentrate on your caring responsibilities and recovery? Ideally, any additional support you look for should be ongoing, rather than a one-off. Getting a cleaner is one such example – they wouldn't be directly tackling your burnout or your caring responsibilities, but they would ease the burden in other areas of your life. Governmental bodies, charities, the voluntary sector and profession-specific bodies can also be a source of support.

Finances

Adulting really can suck, and never more so than when you are horribly burned out but you still need to earn enough to pay the bills and have a decent quality of life. This need has been compounded by the current cost-of-living crisis where our bills, inflation and interest rates have rapidly increased.

You cannot ignore essential costs like your mortgage, bills, childcare, student loan and professional fees. You have to take these into consideration when you are thinking about making changes to your job in burnout.

Dan Bartlett reflects that savings can be useful to dip into during periods of burnout, if you have them:

One practical piece of advice: build up some savings. I have been saved twice (no pun intended) by having enough money saved away to take extended periods off of work. This will not be an option for everyone, but if you can save, it will give you a priceless safety net.

When you're considering your choices post-burnout, if the change that you're considering causes serious financial stress in the medium or long term, it's probably not the right decision for you at this present time. However, not being able to make the changes that you want to immediately because of financial constraints doesn't necessarily mean this will always be the case.

How to Successfully Manage Your Finances During Burnout
Do not bury your head in the sand when it comes to your finances! Otherwise you'll just have another huge stressor in your life, in addition to your work stresses and burnout. Please note, I am not a financial adviser – seek advice from one if this is what you need – but the following tips may be of help to you during burnout:

- Even if you cannot immediately leave your job when you really want to, remember you are likely to have more choice in control than you might think (*see* Exercise 4, p. 42).
- Create a roadmap (*see* p. 161). Can you cut down your hours? Could you develop a portfolio career (*see* p. 157) or set up a business? You might have to think creatively, but hopefully you can plan for a flexible way of working, even if your choices are limited.
- Be ruthless when looking at your outgoings. Are there improvements you can make to your spending to give you some financial flexibility?
- Work out your bottom line – what is the absolute minimum income you can get by on, with a small leeway for unexpected bills?
- Renegotiate with your electricity and gas providers, and see if you could save on insurances and phone contracts to get the best deals you can.
- Avoid unmanageable credit. High interest rates on credit cards and loans and 'buy now pay later' schemes can quickly cause wild debts.
- If you're in over your head, seek expert help sooner rather than later – Citizen's Advice and your bank are good places to start.

Your Role at Work and Your Workplace Itself

Your role at work and the level of seniority or responsibility you have will factor into how easy it will be to make the changes you need to make to your job in order to recover well. Your job contract will also impact on your choices. Some of my colleagues, for instance, are contractually required to work a six-month notice period – and in burnout, this is a long time to stay in a role that is actively harming you. The way to successfully manage this is to write a short-, medium- and long-term plan. Knowing that you are doing small things to move towards your bigger goal will help, even if you can't make changes immediately. (Please refer to the career development section, p. 161, for how to do this practically.)

Finally – and I cannot write a chapter on the things that will prevent you recovering without touching on this – in some workplaces, the burnout culture is so endemic and deeply entrenched that you will not be able to stay well working within them. How you decide to stay or leave will be unique to you, your burnout, the severity of your symptoms and how likely you are to make impactful changes on the factors that caused your burnout, but sometimes the barrier is the workplace itself. (I have talked about this in more depth on p. 54. Feel free to have another read of this section if you identify with this problem.)

Making Difficult Decisions Post-Burnout

We've covered some of the internal and external barriers to a successful recovery from burnout. Now I'm going to help you with the decision-making processes that you'll need to engage with.

In burnout, the decision fatigue is very real, and the amount of energy it takes to make effective decisions feels huge. This is often a barrier to making good, timely decisions post-burnout. If you're able to, please postpone any big decisions after burnout until you have the emotional and mental capacity to make a sound decision. Concentrate on getting better and restoring your health first before exploring your options and facing what is likely to be a series of tough decisions and choices.

You might feel that a decision is hard because:

- the stakes, for you, are particularly high;
- two or more options weigh the same in your mind;
- it brings back unhelpful memories or fears;
- your burnout is directly impacting the decision-making process.

You might go about making a difficult decision using techniques that appear to be rational, such as writing lists of pros and cons, but ultimately decision-making has to come from the heart. We're not rational creatures; a lot of our decisions are based on emotion. When there is a conflict between the head and the heart, decision-making becomes very hard.

You might also become torn between making a decision that feels right for you but falls short of other people's perceived or expressed expectations. Your loved ones, peers and colleagues will all have expectations of your decision-making and you may have commitments that you need to stand by as well.

Another problem with decision-making is that people will offer biased advice, which might not necessarily be right for you, even if it comes from a kind place and is unintentional. This clouds decision-making, rather than making it easier.

Making difficult decisions involves being vulnerable and honest with yourself. But when you embrace the vulnerability and have the courage to make big, brave decisions, then you can let go of any shame or guilt that is associated with those decisions. Ultimately, what defines a difficult decision isn't so much the decision itself but how it is perceived by the decision maker.

How to Make Decisions in Times of Uncertainty

Post-pandemic, it has become even harder to make career decisions because in a lot of sectors and industries, the way we work has changed dramatically and continues to change. Factor in a cost-of-living crisis, economic uncertainty and the emergence of AI (which, although in its early days now, will change the career landscape forever) and your career decisions become much more difficult to make effectively.

When I qualified as a doctor, I knew exactly what being a consultant or a GP would look like when I got there. Now, the nature of the job is changing so rapidly (especially in primary care) that it's difficult to know if it's a job to train for when the way you work at the end of the process is likely to be different than when you started. The careers that we are training for are no longer predictable and the ladder is not necessarily linear – and this isn't just a problem in my industry, either. Everyone is operating in a VUCA (volatile, uncertain, complex and ambiguous) environment. It's hard enough to make effective decisions about your future after burnout, and even harder when living in times of uncertainty and rapid change.

Here are my top tips for making decisions in times of uncertainty:

- Focus on the solvable issues you have, not the things you cannot control, which will lead to frustration.
- Establish habits, routines and predictability in times of uncertainty. Reducing the decision burden eases the mental load. Having routine and predictability in areas of your life that are nothing to do with your work can give you the mental space and capacity to engage in the bigger decisions. Steve Jobs, former CEO of Apple, used to wear the same outfit every day. We've all seen photos of him wearing the black turtleneck sweater, and this was a conscious decision on his part. He said was it was one less decision that he had to make each day and therefore he could focus his attention on the things that really mattered, which was growing his company.
- Accepting uncertainty does not mean not having a plan. In fact, having a plan with flexible and adaptable goals (that bear your values in mind) is helpful for managing uncertainty. Start with small, achievable goals and take baby steps while keeping the long-term plan in the back of your mind.
- Be flexible with your plans and expectations.
- Never make a decision in anger, if you are having mental health problems or if you are early on in burnout recovery. Delay the decision-making in these situations, if possible.

- Always make decisions that align with your values. Honestly, if you don't know which decision to make or direction to go in, trust your values and you really can't go wrong.

Exercise 61

Difficult decisions – journal prompts

The following prompts will help you to make difficult decisions:

- Describe a past decision that you regret. What have you learned from it? How do you feel about it? How is it affecting your current decision-making?
- At the top of the page, write down in one sentence what the difficult decision you're facing is, then jot down every choice you have. Think of as many options as possible. Remember that not making a decision is also a decision.
- For each option, write down what your initial gut reaction is to that choice and why.
- Imagine that you pick each option. Visualise your life in five years' time – what does it look like after making each choice? Write as much as you can for each option.
- Write down whether each choice aligns with or brings you closer to your values (*see* p. 144). If not, why not?
- Look at each choice. Does it make you feel energised or drained?
- Hopefully by now it will be more obvious which choice is right for you. Pick the one that appears to be calling to you. What information or support do you need to help you feel more comfortable with this choice?

Final thoughts

We have now come to the end of this guide but, for some of you, this is likely to be just the beginning of overcoming burnout.

For those of you that started this book knowing that you were working in a high-stress job, I hope that you have come away with insight, knowledge and strategies for effectively preventing a worsening of any burnout risk. With the tools provided, you now have a much higher chance of being able to successfully avoid burning out.

For those of you that started this book wondering whether you are burned out, I hope that you have been able to get some clarity on where you're at, as well as gaining valuable knowledge about what you really need to do, both in the short and long term, to effectively recover.

For those of you that started this book part way through recovery, or if you were wondering why your recovery was not going as well or as quickly as you'd expected, I hope that you'll now have clarity on the things that need to be done differently, and that you feel reassured in knowing what to do next.

For those of you that started reading this book because you were worried about a friend, colleague or loved one, I hope you now have an insight into how and why this person is acting the way they are and how you can effectively support them through their burnout.

Regardless of where you're at with burnout, and irrespective of your motivation for reading this book, you'll know that staying well in the context of high levels of stress is difficult. Effective burnout prevention and recovery is sadly not as simple or straightforward as doing a bit more yoga or meditation. However, with this book you will now be empowered to identify the root cause of any of your work stressors.

You'll also have a much better idea about how and where to spend your limited energy in making evidence-based changes that will really move the needle for you.

If you are now embarking on a recovery journey, I'm sure you will be aware that staying well after burnout is a huge challenge. The temptation to slip back into old patterns of behaviour at work will be huge, particularly if you're not supported to maintain the crucial changes you've implemented to stay well. This lack of support might come from other people, organisations or systems, but similarly, it's also all too easy to fall back into previous ways of coping with stress, and become overwhelmed again.

You've already had a head start on ensuring that your recovery journey is successful, because you've read this book! Even with this knowledge, there will be moments along the way that feel really hard, but please be reassured that it will get easier. It might take many months, even years, but burnout is not a permanent problem. In going through the recovery process steps you will start to feel better. Hang on in there!

In this book I have given you everything I know from my own lived experience of burnout, coupled with over 20 years of clinical knowledge, experience and my background in neuroscience. Burnout is the hardest thing I have ever had to overcome, but just over two years after being discharged from Practitioner Health, and coming up to five years after my initial burnout crisis, I'm fairly confident in saying that I have – so far – managed to sustain my recovery. I know that the changes I've made will keep me on an even keel.

My Recovery Milestones

To finish, I want to touch on some of the milestones that I experienced during this recovery period. As I've said, recovery is long and often tough, but reaching recovery milestones is a great opportunity for you to reflect and realise just how far you've come. Some of my milestones were about big changes that happened to my behaviour, such as improving my self-neglect habits; others were incredibly personal and deeply meaningful, such as Milestone 2; but the majority were simply breakthroughs in how I felt.

These milestones were all things that were significant to me in demonstrating that I had made progress, but what you consider to be significant might well be different to my own experience. Therefore, you might ask how you know when you reach a milestone. Trust me when I say that you'll just *know* when you've made significant progress to have reached a milestone. I've put my milestones in chronological order, so that you can see how I progressed over the months and years.

Milestone 1

At the height of my burnout I often struggled to find the energy to shower, clean my teeth or wash my face. Starting to look after myself and prioritising self-care was one of the first big milestones that I achieved in my recovery. (I'm not talking about self-care in the superficial, glossy wellness aesthetic it has become on social media, I'm talking the basics, such as getting dressed, eating something and washing my face.) Being quite truthful, I only did these things at the start because my husband made me accountable. But doing these acts of basic self-care was a huge accomplishment and a crucial first step to dragging myself out of the dark hole I was in.

Milestone 2

The next significant milestone in my recovery was during a mundane, insignificant outing with my children. I don't even remember what we were doing, but I do remember how I felt. My burnout made me very depressed and I'd felt flat, hopeless and unmotivated for a long period of time, but on this outing I suddenly had a moment of realisation that I was enjoying myself. I hadn't experienced genuine enjoyment for so long that the novelty and force of the sensation hit me hard. It was as if I'd gone from seeing everything in black and white to vivid colour, such was the difference.

This was significant because I'd become so lost in the despondency of burnout that I'd forgotten what it felt like to be happy. I remember welling up, feeling overwhelmed and angry that my burnout had robbed me of enjoying time with my children while they were still very young, but I was also extremely grateful that I could feel something good again.

Milestone 3

The realisation that there were more good days than bad was a big milestone. It took months to get there, but it was a huge relief when I experienced it. I was able to consciously recognise it because I was being proactive about monitoring my stress levels. (Flick back to p. 196 for ideas on how to monitor your stress levels going forward!)

Milestone 4

Going back to NHS work after my second burnout and being able to successfully manage my work stress was a huge milestone. (I've written about the moment when I realised that I could return to work and successfully manage my stress levels back on p. 199.) I was so worried about my return, but it felt so good to be back in an environment where I knew I would be subject to stress and I could use the techniques I'd learned in therapy to keep myself well.

Milestone 5

Having the energy, concentration and focus to start being proactive (rather than reactive) about my well-being and needs was a big milestone. This began by asking for help as needed (and accepting it, too – a game changer for a people pleaser like me). I started to proactively look after my well-being by joining a gym and actually going to classes. I also scheduled all of the dental, optician and medical appointments I'd been putting off. Around this time, I also started reading for pleasure again – this was a wonderful milestone to achieve, especially as I am a massive bookworm!

Milestone 6

One of the enduring symptoms during my recovery was the most incredible fatigue. In the early days of returning to NHS work, I'd do a four- or six-hour shift and then spend the next day on the sofa, physically and emotionally drained to empty. With time, the severity of my fatigue decreased, as did the amount of time I needed to spend on the sofa after work. Getting back to doing a full day's work (with significant changes made, of course!) without the need for prolonged rest after was a huge recovery milestone for me.

Milestone 7

The realisation that my ability to problem solve effectively was back to pre-burnout levels was a wonderful milestone, but one that took quite a long time to come back.

Milestone 8

The very last thing that came back, about four years or so after my first burnout, was my confidence. Getting a place on the NHS Clinical Entrepreneur Programme and having my eyes opened to the world of entrepreneurship and start-ups was the thing that really moved the needle on my confidence levels. It came at the perfect time when I was recovered enough to really make the most of the opportunities that arose as a result of being on this programme.

As a direct result of being on this programme, I went on to co-found a start-up and work on it full-time. This demonstrated to me that I could work hard – with boundaries in place – and juggle multiple demands successfully. There was a point where I didn't think I would have the energy or capacity to work full-time again, but I then knew that I could do it.

What's more, even though my first start-up didn't work out, this time my mindset over the failure was completely different to my mindset during burnout. While my confidence levels are something that I still intermittently struggle with, it is wonderful to feel confident in myself again. I have learned so much about myself, my abilities and my strengths, and I'm a world apart from where I was five years ago.

My Post-Burnout Career

Now, I am flourishing. My post-burnout career is very different to the career I thought I would have pre-burnout, but I am 100 per cent here for it! I am still a practising doctor, but my career goals are now slightly different. Instead of being pulled to clinical practice, I am drawn to helping other doctors create medical careers that are sustainable, and I am exploring my options within HealthTech start-ups, where I can take my clinical knowledge and experience and apply it to products and solutions that will impact at scale. I have successfully created a unique career portfolio that allows me to pursue my passions of mental health education and advocacy through education, coaching, mentoring, digital products and public speaking.

At the start of my post-burnout career, there was no way that I could have anticipated being in the position I am right now. I began my recovery process making career decisions out of necessity and survival. I had to grieve for the career I thought I was going to have. But, where I am now is even better than what I had hoped or planned for pre-burnout. While every post-burnout career journey is different, it is possible to find your way and to find fulfilment, even in unexpected places. The exercises I've shared will help you to get there too.

It took several years, but I can finally say that the old Claire is back. I'll likely carry the scars for some time, but I think I can say that I'm there now. It's taken a lot of hard, deep work to do it, but I've done it. I hope in sharing my milestones that I can give a bit of hope to anyone that is currently experiencing the absolute pit of despair that is burnout right now. You can and will get better. You've absolutely got this.

Parting advice

If you take nothing else away from this book, these are the key things to remember!

- Prevention is better than cure, so if you are able to catch yourself before you reach burnout it will be easier to make successful changes to manage your stress levels.
- You might have individual risk factors that put you at risk of burnout, but by definition, burnout is a workplace problem. It occurs at the extreme end of your body's normal reaction to prolonged stress.
- You can do all the work on your stress-management skills and coping techniques, but if your workplace is still a difficult place you will burn out again. So, you must ensure that you make changes to the root cause of your workplace stress. Some will be able to do this successfully without leaving their jobs, but for others this might mean having to leave. But remember, burnout recovery does not necessarily mean needing to make drastic changes.
- Recovery is multifaceted, but if you concentrate on nothing else, make it these three things: regaining control at work (in whatever form that takes for you), regaining control over your well-being and having supportive relationships.
- Recovery is not linear. Not every bad day means you're sliding again, but if those bad days become more persistent or if your symptoms of burnout are getting worse, then early intervention is crucial. Having said that, don't sweat the bad days; they don't necessarily mean the burnout's coming back. Stay calm, breathe, make space, don't panic.

- You're not the only one that has experienced this awfulness, but burnout is a horribly isolating experience and it will often feel that you're the only person in this position. Reach out, find a community that will support you – and use them!
- Respect your burnout. Recovery is slow because of the huge number that burnout does on your brain and body. Your new normal will be frustrating beyond belief, but you cannot rush things. Follow the process of recovery, and things will fall into place with time.
- Recovery has to focus on changing – or effectively managing – the root cause of your stress.
- You will have to do some pretty hard sh*t during your recovery, and you will have to make some difficult decisions about the changes that need to happen to stay well. Truthfully, anyone that gets through burnout is a resilient badass. You are incredible and you will get there.
- The process is hard, so remember to hold yourself with the compassion and kindness that you so dearly deserve.
- Don't fret about the opinions of people that haven't been through burnout, because (luckily for them!) they just won't be able to truly understand what it is to experience it. As Brené Brown famously said in one of her talks, 'If you're not in the arena also getting your ass kicked, I'm not interested in your feedback'!
- Burnout is not a permanent state of being. You *can* and *will* feel better, hang on in there because better days are coming. It won't feel like it in the depths, but you will be a better person with a better career because of what you've gone through. You will have more appreciation of the things that really matter to you, and you will come out with more clarity on your purpose, values and direction. With this book, you now have the skills and the knowledge to create better ways of working and living. There is hope and so much to look forward to.

I wish you all the best going forward.

References

Introduction

'A whopping 91 per cent'
Mental Health UK, *The Burnout Report* (January 2024), https://euc7zxtct58
.exactdn.com/wp-content/uploads/2024/01/19145241/Mental-Health-UK
_The-Burnout-Report-2024.pdf

Chapter 1

'... first described in the 1970s by a psychologist'
Freudenberger, H. J., 'Staff Burn-Out', *Journal of Social Issues*, 30 (Winter 1974),
pp. 159–65, https://doi.org/10.1111/j.1540-4560.1974.tb00706.x
'An occupational syndrome that arises as a result of prolonged workplace stress that has not been successfully managed.'
World Health Organization, 'Burn-out an "Occupational Phenomenon":
International Classification of Diseases' (28 May, 2019), www.who.int/news
/item/28-05-2019-burn-out-an-occupational-phenomenon-international
-classification-of-diseases
'Most commonly, people suffering with burnout first start experiencing "emotional exhaustion"'
Taris, T. W. and Schaufeli W. B., 'The Job Demands-Resources Model', *The Wiley Blackwell Handbook of the Psychology of Occupational Safety and Workplace Health* (October 2015), https://doi.org/10.1002/9781118979013.ch8
'... the physical symptoms of burnout'
Salvagioni, D. A. G., et al. 'Physical, Psychological and Occupational Consequences of Job Burnout: A systematic review of prospective studies', PLoS One, 12(10) (4 Oct 2017), https://doi.org/10.1371/journal.pone.0185781
'For people with an adaptive stress response'
Oosterholt, B. G., Maes, J. H., Van der Linden, D., et al. 'Burnout and Cortisol: Evidence for a lower cortisol awakening response in both clinical and

nonclinical burnout', *Journal of Psychosomatic Research*, 78 (May 2015), pp. 445–51, DOI: 10.1016/j.jpsychores.2014.11.003

'... *20 per cent increased risk of atrial fibrillation*'

Garg P. K., Claxton J. S., Soliman E. Z., et al. 'Associations of Anger, Vital Exhaustion, Anti-depressant Use, and Poor Social Ties with Incident Atrial Fibrillation: The atherosclerosis risk in communities study', *Eur J Prev Cardiol.*, (2020), DOI: 10.1177/2047487319897163

'... *employees scoring in the top 20 per cent on the burnout scale at baseline had a whopping 79 per cent increased risk of being diagnosed with coronary heart disease over a three-year period*'

Toker, S., Melamed, S., Berliner, S., et al. 'Burnout and Risk of Coronary Heart Disease: A prospective study of 8838 employees', *Psychosomatic Medicine*, 74 (October 2012), pp. 840–847, DOI: 10.1097/PSY.0b013e31826c3174

'*Researchers think that the altered stress response is one of the causes*'

Melamed, S., Ugarten, U., Shirom, A., et al. 'Chronic Burnout, Somatic Arousal and Elevated Salivary Cortisol Levels', *J Psychosom Res.*, 46(6) (June 1999), pp. 59–98, DOI: 10.1016/s0022-3999(99)00007-0

'*56 per cent of burned-out doctors reported changing food habits*'

Barello S., Palamenghi L. and Graffigna G., 'Burnout and Somatic Symptoms Among Frontline Healthcare Professionals at the Peak of the Italian COVID-19 Pandemic', *Psychiatry Res.*, 290 (August 2020), DOI: 10.1016/j.psychres.2020.113129

'*If you are under the age of 45 and you burn out, you have an increased risk of dying prematurely from any cause*'

Salvagioni, D. A. G., et al. 'Physical, Psychological and Occupational Consequences of Job Burnout: A systematic review of prospective studies', *PLoS One*, 12(10) (4 October, 2017), https://doi.org/10.1371/journal.pone.0185781

'*Let's start by talking about some of the psychological symptoms of burnout*'

Koutsimani, P., Montgomery, A., Masoura, E. and Panagopoulou, E. 'Burnout and Cognitive Performance', *Int J Environ Res Public Health*, 18(4): 2145 (22 February, 2021), DOI: 10.3390/ijerph18042145.

'*Poor memory*'

Deligkaris, P., Panagopoulou, E., Montgomery, A. J. and Masoura, E., 'Job Burnout and Cognitive Functioning: A systematic review', *Work & Stress*, 28 (13 March 2014), pp. 107–23, DOI: 10.1080/02678373.2014.909545

'*If you're interested in the detailed science behind these psychological symptoms, then here's the geeky bit*'

Savic, I., 'Structural Changes of the Brain in Relation to Occupational Stress', *Cerebral Cortex*, 25 (2015), pp. 1554–64, DOI: 10.1093/cercor/bht348

'... *such as post-traumatic stress disorder*'

Morey R. A., Gold A. L., LaBar K. S., et al., 'Amygdala Volume Changes in Posttraumatic Stress Disorder in a Large Case-Controlled Veterans Group',

Arch Gen Psychiatry, 69(11) (November 2012), pp. 1169–78, DOI: 10.1001/archgenpsychiatry.2012.50

'*In lab studies, the brains of stressed rats return to normal structure and function when stress is removed*'
Liston, C., McEwen, B. S. and Casey, B. J., 'Psychosocial Stress Reversibly Disrupts Prefrontal Processing and Attentional Control', *Proceedings of the National Academy of Sciences*, 106 (2009), pp. 912–17, DOI: 10.1073/pnas.0807041106

'*... has been found to reduce the size of the amygdala and return the prefrontal cortex to normal*'
Savic, I., 'Structural Changes of the Brain in Relation to Occupational Stress', *Cerebral Cortex*, 25 (2015), pp. 1554–64, DOI: 10.1093/cercor/bht348

'*... useful in the treatment of burnout*'
Frögéli, E., Djordjevic, A., Rudman, A., et al. 'A Randomized Controlled Pilot Trial of Acceptance and Commitment Training (ACT) for Preventing Stress-Related Ill Health among Future Nurses', *Anxiety Stress Coping*, 29(2) (2016), pp. 202–18, DOI: 10.1080/10615806.2015.1025765

'*Around 60 per cent of people with burnout have a concurrent mental health problem, like anxiety or depression*'
Koutsimani, P., Montgomery, A. and Georganta, K., 'The Relationship Between Burnout, Depression, and Anxiety: A systematic review and meta-analysis', *Frontiers in Psychology*, 10 (13 March, 2019), https://doi.org/10.3389/fpsyg.2019.00284

'*Generalised anxiety*'
The National Institute of Clinical Excellence, 'Diagnosis of Generalized Anxiety Disorder' (February 2024), https://cks.nice.org.uk/topics/generalized-anxiety-disorder/diagnosis/diagnosis

'*When screening for depression, a doctor might ask the following questions*'
The National Institute for Clinical Excellence, 'Depression: When Should I Suspect a Diagnosis of Depression?' (April 2024), https://cks.nice.org.uk/topics/depression/diagnosis/diagnosis

'*... around 40 per cent of workers with burnout are prescribed antidepressant medication*'
Walker, L., '"Too Much Too Quickly": 40 per cent of burnout patients given antidepressants', *The Brussels Times* (28 October, 2021), www.brusselstimes.com/190980/too-much-too-quickly-40-of-burnout-patients-given-antidepressants

'*having burnout means you are more likely to be prescribed antidepressants*'
Madsen, I. E. H., et al, 'Burnout as a Risk Factor for Antidepressant Treatment – A repeated measures time-to-event analysis of 2936 Danish human service workers', *Journal of Psychiatric Research*, 65 (June 2015), pp. 47–52, https://doi.org/10.1016/j.jpsychires.2015.04.004

Chapter 2

'These six factors are...'
Maslach, C. and Leiter, M. P., 'Understanding the Burnout Experience: Recent research and its implications for psychiatry', *World Psychiatry*, 15(2) (5 June 2016), pp. 103–11, DOI: 10.1002/wps.20311

'Circle of control'
Developed by Covey S. R., *The 7 Habits of Highly Effective People: Powerful lessons in personal change* (Simon and Schuster, 2004)

'... women effectively work two months of every year for free as compared to their male counterparts'
Office for National Statistics, *Gender Pay Gap in the UK, 2022* (October 2022), www.ons.gov.uk/employmentandlabourmarket/peopleinwork/earning sandworkinghours/bulletins/genderpaygapintheuk/2022

'... women hospital doctors still earn on average 18.9 per cent less than men based on a comparison of full-time equivalent mean pay'
NHS Resolution, *2021 Gender Pay Gap Report* (October 2021), https://resolution .nhs.uk/wp-content/uploads/2022/03/Gender-Pay-Gap-Report-2021.pdf

'... 20 per cent of your time at work doing personally meaningful work in order to reduce your burnout risk by half'
Shanafelt, T. D., West, C. P., Sloan J. A., et al., 'Career Fit and Burnout Among Academic Faculty', *Arch Intern Med*, 169(10) (2009), pp. 990–95, DOI: 10.1001/archinternmed.2009.70

'the Motivation-Hygiene Theory'
Originally described in the 1950s by Frederick Herzberg, and discussed here: Bassett-Jones, N. and Lloyd, G. C., 'Does Herzberg's Motivation Theory Have Staying Power?' *Journal of Management Development*, 24 (1 December, 2005), pp. 929–43, DOI: 10.1108/02621710510627064

'Positive social support, i.e. sharing and celebrating successes within the team'
Rieckert, A., et al. 'How Can We Build and Maintain the Resilience of Our Health Care Professionals During COVID-19? Recommendations Based on a Scoping Review', *BMJ Open*, 11(1) (6 January, 2011), DOI: 10.1136/ bmjopen-2020-043718

Chapter 3

'70 per cent of people experience some degree of imposter syndrome'
Sakullu, J. and Alexander, J., 'The Imposter Phenomenon', *International Journal of Behavioral Science*, 6(1) (2011), pp. 75–97

'... seemingly confident individuals, such as Michelle Obama, have admitted to having imposter syndrome.'

BBC News, 'Michelle Obama: "I still have impostor syndrome"' (4 December, 2018), www.bbc.co.uk/news/uk-46434147

'Over time, this leads to excessive workload and burnout'

Hewitt, P. L. and Flett, G. L., 'Perfectionism in the Self and Social Contexts: Conceptualization, assessment, and association with psychopathology'. *Journal of Personality and Social Psychology*, 60(3) (March 1991), pp. 456–70. DOI: 10.1037/0022-3514.60.3.456

'Perfectionism can directly cause reduced job satisfaction and burnout'

Chen, W. and Li, Y., 'Perfectionism, Job Satisfaction, and Burnout Among Chinese Nurses: A moderated mediation model', *Journal of Occupational Health Psychology*, 26(2) (2021), pp. 191–203, DOI: 10.1037/ocp0000238

'... may take on too much work or have a hard time saying no to requests from colleagues, which can lead to burnout due to excessive workload and emotional exhaustion'

Lee, R. T. and Ashforth, B. E., 'A Meta-Analytic Examination of the Correlates of the Three Dimensions of Job Burnout', *Journal of Occupational Health Psychology*, 1(2) (April 1996), pp. 111–27, DOI: 10.1037/0021-9010.81.2.123

'Write your own Bill of Personal Rights'

Bourne, E. J., *The Anxiety and Phobia Workbook*, 4th Edition (New Harbinger Publications, 2005)

'Your personality type might very well put you at increased risk of burnout' and *'extroversion appears to be protective against burnout'*

Angelini, G., 'Big Five Model Personality Traits and Job Burnout: A systematic literature review', *BMC Psychol,* 11(49) (19 February, 2023), https://doi.org/10.1186/s40359-023-01056-y

'The key point here in determining whether an introvert is more at risk of burnout or not is the type of job that is being done'

Psychology, 'Person-Environment Fit', http://psychology.iresearchnet.com/industrial-organizational-psychology/recruitment/person-environment-fit

'This in turn directly affects your risk of burnout as an adult'

Lam, C. B. and Tang, C. S., 'The Effects of Parental Control and Interpersonal Behavior on the Development of Work Stress: The mediation role of achievement motivation', *Journal of Vocational Behavior*, 62(2) (2003), pp. 213–29, DOI: 10.1016/S0001-8791(02)00040-9

'ACEs can increase your burnout risk as an adult'

Rospenda, K. M., Richman, J. A. and Shannon, C. A., 'Prevalence and Mental Health Correlates of Harassment and Discrimination in the Workplace: Results from a national study', *International Journal of Stress Management*, 16(3) (2009), pp. 205–26, DOI: 10.1037/a0016539

'Exposure to traumatic events as an adult'

Prati, G., Pietrantoni, L. and Cicognani, E., 'Coping Strategies and Collective Efficacy as Moderators of the Relationship Between Stressors and Burnout

Among Emergency Medical Rescuers', *Journal of Traumatic Stress,* 23(2) (2010), pp. 1–9, https://doi.org/10.1037/2157-3905.1.S.84

'PTSD, which can develop after exposure to a traumatic event, also puts individuals at a higher risk of burnout'

Marshall, G. N., Schell, T. L., Miles, J. N. V. and Pintaric, T., 'Determinants of PTSD Symptom Severity and Functional Impairment Among Veterans Seeking Help for Posttraumatic Stress Disorder', *Journal of Occupational Health Psychology,* 18(3) (2013), pp. 275–87, DOI: 10.1037/a0032859.

'... directly linked to burnout are anxiety'

Dahlin, M., Joneborg, N. and Runeson, B., 'Stress and Depression Among Medical Students: A cross-sectional study', *Medical Education,* 39(6) (June 2005), pp. 594–604, DOI: 10.1111/j.1365-2929.2005.02176.x

'... and depression'

Shirom, A. and Melamed, S., 'A Comparison of the Construct Validity of Two Burnout Measures in Two Groups of Professionals', *International Journal of Stress Management,* 13(2) (2006), pp. 176–200, DOI: 10.1037/1072-5245.13.2.176

'... substance misuse problems, such as alcohol or recreational drugs'

Finn, P. R., Kivlahan, D. R. and Huggins, G. R., 'Burnout Among Working Women: A study of occupational and personal stressors', *Journal of Addictive Diseases,* 14(2) (1995), pp. 103–18, DOI: 10.1300/J069v14n02_09

'... it helps to move towards problem-focused coping styles'

Maslach, C. and Leiter, M. P., 'Understanding Burnout: New Models' in C. L. Cooper and J. C. Quick (eds.), *The Handbook of Stress and Health: A guide to research and practice* (John Wiley & Sons, 2016), pp. 37–50

'Self-efficacy is an individual's belief in their ability to perform a task or achieve a goal'

Stoeber, J. and Janssen, D. P., 'Perfectionism and Coping with Daily Failures: Positive reframing helps achieve satisfaction at the end of the day', *Anxiety, Stress, & Coping,* 24(5) (October 2011), pp. 477–97, DOI: 10.1080/10615806.2011.562977

'Some emotional coping styles (such as denial and avoidance) are associated with higher levels of burnout'

Lazarus, R. S. and Folkman, S., *Stress, Appraisal and Coping* (Springer Publishing Company, 1984)

'ADHD in adulthood might look like'

Adapted from the 'Adult ADHD Self-Report Scale (ASRS-v1.1) Symptom Checklist', www.hcp.med.harvard.edu/ncs/ftpdir/adhd/18Q_ASRS_English.pdf

'... difficulties with time management, organisational skills and stress management'

Barkley, R. A., Murphy, K. R. and Fischer, M., *ADHD in Adults: What the Science Says* (Guilford Press, 2008)

'Autistic burnout is conceptualised as resulting from chronic life stress and a mismatch of expectations and abilities without adequate support'

Raymaker, D., 'Understanding Autistic Burnout', *National Autistic Society* (1 March, 2022), www.autism.org.uk/advice-and-guidance/professional-practice/autistic-burnout

'*People with ADHD take significantly more stress-related days off sick than those that do not have ADHD*'

De Graaf, R., Kessler, R. C., Fayyad J., et al., 'The Prevalence and Effects of Adult Attention-Deficit/Hyperactivity Disorder (ADHD) on the Performance of Workers: Results from the WHO World Mental Health Survey Initiative', *Occup Environ Med*, 65 (2008), pp. 835–42, https://doi.org/10.1136/oem.2007.038448

'*CBT can help with...*'

Multiple studies, as outlined here: https://div12.org/treatment/cognitive -behavioral-therapy-for-adult-adhd

'*... inattention is a stronger predictor of burnout than hyperactivity*'

Combs, M. A., Canu, W. H., Broman-Fulks, J. J., et al., 'Perceived Stress and ADHD Symptoms in Adults', *J Atten Disord*, 19 (2015), pp. 425–34, https://doi .org/10.1177/1087054712459558

'*Regular mindfulness exercises reduce inattentiveness, hyperactivity and impulsivity in people with ADHD*'

Cairncross, M. and Miller, C. J., 'The Effectiveness of Mindfulness-Based Therapies for ADHD: A meta-analytic review', *Journal of Attention Disorders*, 24(5) (2020), pp. 627–43

'*... doing flow/meditative activities such as yoga and Tai Chi are just as beneficial*'

Zhang, Z., Chang, X., Zhang, W., et al., 'The Effect of Meditation-based Mind-Body Interventions on Symptoms and Executive Function in People With ADHD: A meta-analysis of randomized controlled trials', *Journal of Attention Disorders*, 27(6) (2023), pp. 583–97, https://doi.org/10.1177/10870547231154897

'*Parents and caregivers*'

Abramson, A., 'The Impact of Parental Burnout', *American Psychological Association* (1 October, 2021), www.apa.org/monitor/2021/10/cover-parental -burnout

'*... any intervention that focuses solely on the individual (such as mindfulness techniques) alone*'

Malik, H. and Annabi, C. A., 'The Impact of Mindfulness Practice on Physician Burnout: A scoping review', *Front Psychol.* (20 September, 2022), DOI: 10.3389/fpsyg.2022.956651

'*... mothers are 28 per cent more likely than fathers to burn out*'

Maven, 'Parents are the Best Workplaces: The largest-ever study of working parents' (2020), https://info.mavenclinic.com/pdf/parents-at-the-best-work-places?submissionGuid=706cbe04-fc38-4089-8740-76d21d0533ce

'*... women do more of the household chores compared to men*'

US Bureau of Labor Statistics, 'Economic News Release' (2008), www.bls.gov/ news.release/atus2.t01.htm

'*This disproportionate share of the mental workload is associated with a poorer sense of well-being for women*'

Ciciolla, L. and Luthar, S. S., 'Invisible Household Labor and Ramifications for Adjustment: Mothers as captains of households', *Sex Roles*, 81(7–8) (2019), pp. 467–86, DOI:10.1007/s11199-018-1001-x

'Women are much more likely to handle the other steps in the process'
Daminger, A., 'The Cognitive Dimension of Household Labor', *American Sociological Review*, 84(4) (2019), pp. 609–33, https://doi.org/10.1177/0003122419859007
'... moderate to severe impact on workplace productivity and increased absenteeism rates'
Ponzo S., et al., 'Menstrual Cycle-associated Symptoms and Workplace Productivity in US Employees: A cross-sectional survey of users of the Flo mobile phone app', *Digit Health* 8 (15 December, 2022), DOI: 10.1177/20552076221145852

Chapter 4

'Five stages of burnout'
As adapted from the 12 stages of burnout, first described by Freudenberger H. J., 'Counseling and Dynamics: Treating the end-stage person', in: Jones J. W. (ed.), *The Burnout Syndrome: Current research, theory, interventions* (London House Press, 1982)
'... abbreviated Burnout Assessment Tool'
Schaufeli, W. B., De Witte, H. and Desart, S., 'Manual Burnout Assessment Tool (BAT)' (July 2020), https://burnoutassessmenttool.be/wp-content/uploads/2020/08/Test-Manual-BAT-English-version-2.0-1.pdf

Part III: Recovery From Burnout: Your Six-Step Recovery Plan

'... six steps of burnout recovery'
Bernier, D., 'A Study of Coping: Successful recovery from severe burnout and other reactions to severe work-related stress', *Work & Stress*, 12(1) (January 1998), pp. 50–65, https://doi.org/10.1080/02678379808256848
'... a change of workplace or job has not been found to be a decisive factor when it comes to a successful recovery period'
Salminen, S., Mäkikangas, A., Hätinen, M., et al., 'My Well-Being In My Own Hands: Experiences of beneficial recovery during burnout rehabilitation', *J Occup Rehabil.*, 25 (May 2015), pp. 733–41, https://doi.org/10.1007/s10926-015-9581-6
'Good relationships'
Hald G. M., Ciprić A., Strizzi J. M. and Sander S., '"Divorce Burnout" Among Recently Divorced Individuals', *Stress and Health*, 36 (March 2020), pp. 457–68, https://doi.org/10.1002/smi.2940

'... effort-recovery theory'
Meijman, T. F. and Mulder, G., 'Psychological Aspects of Workload' in P. J. D. Drenth, H. Thierry and C. J. de Wolff (eds.), A *Handbook of Work and Organizational Psychology: Work Psychology* (Psychology, 1998)
'... the more we're struggling with our health'
Sonnentag, S., 'The Recovery Paradox: Portraying the complex interplay between job stressors, lack of recovery, and poor well-being', *Research in Organizational Behavior*, 38 (2018), pp. 169–85, https://doi.org/10.1016/j.riob.2018.11.002
'... the severity of your burnout will determine how well you respond to these measures'
Oerlemans W. G. and Bakker A. B., 'Burnout and Daily Recovery: A day reconstruction study', *J Occup Health Psychol.*, 19(3) (July 2014), pp. 303–14, DOI: 10.1037/a0036904
'Identifying unhelpful styles of thinking'
Multiple researchers and iterations, as outlined in: 'Cognitive Distortions – Unhelpful Thinking Styles (Extended)', www.psychologytools.com/resource/cognitive-distortions-unhelpful-thinking-styles-extended
'...one common thing that happens to everyone that experiences burnout'
Bernier, D., 'A Study of Coping: Successful recovery from severe burnout and other reactions to severe work-related stress', *Work & Stress*, 12(1) (January 1998), pp. 50–65, https://doi.org/10.1080/02678379808256848
'Job crafting means taking proactive steps to redesign what you do at work'
Tims, M. and Bakker, A. B., 'Job Crafting: Towards a new model of individual job redesign', *South African Journal of Industrial Psychology*, 36 (2010), pp. 1–9, https://doi.org/10.4102/sajip.v36i2.841
'The idea of job crafting is to empower you to have control over your career'
Multiple studies, summarised and accessed here: www.sciencedirect.com/topics/psychology/job-crafting
'There are three ways to job craft'
Berg, J. M., Dutton, J. E. and Wrzesniewski, A., 'Job Crafting and Meaningful Work', in B. J. Dik, Z. S. Byrne and M. F. Steger (eds.), *Purpose and Meaning in the Workplace* (American Psychological Association, 2013), pp. 81–104, https://doi.org/10.1037/14183-005
'I've seen portfolio careers described as "squiggly careers", and this description is pretty spot on'
Tupper, H. and Ellis S., *The Squiggly Career* (Portfolio Penguin, 2020)
'Higher than average income'
The Centre for Research on Self-Employment (CRSE), accessed via www.ipse.co.uk/policy/research/crse.html
'SMART goals in ACT look like'
Adapted from: www.actmindfully.com.au/upimages/Goal_Setting_Worksheet.pdf
'The seven Rs for lasting change'
Harris, R., 'The Top Tools for Lasting Change – Part 1' (24 May, 2018), www.thehappinesstrap.com/top-tools-lasting-change-part-1

'... daily recovery efforts are more important and effective than waiting for the weekend or a less-frequent but longer annual holiday' and '... it's smartphone use, in particular, that will hamper your recovery'

Derks, D. and Bakker, A. B., 'Smartphone Use, Work–Home Interference, and Burnout: A diary study on the role of recovery', *Applied Psychology: An International Review*, 63(3) (2014), pp. 411–440, https://doi.org/10.1111/j.1464-0597.2012.00530.x

'While holidays might help you feel temporarily better, their effects are not maintained on return'

Etzion, D., 'Annual Vacation: Duration of relief from job stressors and burnout', *Anxiety, Stress, and Coping*, 16 (22 May, 2003), pp. 213–26, https://doi.org/10.1080/10615806.2003.10382974

'The Pomodoro® Technique'

Developed by Francesco Cirillo, accessed from: https://www.pomodorotechnique

'... completing the stress cycle'

Nagoski E. and Nagoski A., *Burnout: The Secret to Unlocking the Stress Cycle* (Vermilion, 2020)

'... learning or mastering a new skill outside of work can help with recovery'

Ginoux, C., Isoard-Gautheur, S. and Sarrazin, P., '"What Did You Do This Weekend?" Relationships between weekend activities, recovery experiences, and changes in work-related well-being', *Applied Psychology Health and Well-Being*, 13 (17 April, 2021), https://doi.org/10.1111/aphw.12272

'... flow state, when you're so engrossed in a task that you lose sense of time passing by'

Aust, F., Beneke, T., Peifer, C. and Wekenborg, M., 'The Relationship Between Flow Experience and Burnout Symptoms: A systematic review', *Int J Environ Res Public Health*, 19(7) (24 March, 2022), 3865, DOI: 10.3390/ijerph19073865

'helpful technique for managing your anxiety and depression and reducing stress'

Multiple studies, summarised and accessed from: https://positivepsychology.com/benefits-of-journaling

'A cognitive bias is a systemic error that occurs in thinking when people are processing and interpreting information about the world around them'

Multiple studies; a comprehensive summary is available here: www.sciencedirect.com/topics/neuroscience/cognitive-bias

'The sunk cost fallacy describes the tendency to follow through on a decision if we have already invested time, effort or money into it, regardless of whether or not the current costs outweigh the benefits'

Arkes H. A. and Blumer, C., 'The Psychology of Sunk Cost', *Organizational Behavior and Human Decision* Processes, 35(1) (1985), pp. 124–40, https://doi.org/10.1016/0749-5978(85)90049-4

'commitment bias describes our tendency to remain committed to our past behaviours and choices'

Schwenk, C. R., 'Information, Cognitive Biases, and Commitment to a Course of Action', *The Academy of Management Review*, 11(2) (1986), pp. 298–310, https://doi.org/10.2307/258461

'... people actually have more respect for those that are able to admit that something's gone wrong'

Chiu, C.-Y. (Chad), Balkundi, P., Owens, B. P. and Tesluk, P. E., 'Shaping Positive and Negative Ties to Improve Team Effectiveness: The roles of leader humility and team helping norms', *Human Relations*, 75(3) (6 November, 2020), pp. 502–31, https://doi.org/10.1177/0018726720968135

'Choice overload is also known as the paradox of choice' and *'When people go into shops with the intention of browsing'*

Chernev, A., Böckenholt, U. and Goodman, J., 'Choice Overload: A conceptual review and meta-analysis', *Journal of Consumer Psychology*, 25(2) (29 August, 2014), pp. 333–58, https://doi.org/10.1016/j.jcps.2014.08.002

'Status quo bias refers to our innate preference as human beings for the current state of affairs'

Samuelson, W. and Zeckhauser, R., 'Status Quo Bias in Decision Making', *Journal of Risk and Uncertainty*, 1(1) (March 1988), pp. 7–59, www.jstor.org/stable/41760530

'In a fixed mindset, you believe that your intelligence and talents are fixed and static'

Yeager, D. S., et al., 'A National Experiment Reveals Where a Growth Mindset Improves Achievement', *Nature* 573 (2019), pp. 364–69, https://doi.org/10.1038/s41586-019-1466-y

'... the experience of guilt is linked so closely to burnout that it has been speculated that it should be added to its symptoms and definition'

Figueiredo-Ferraz H., et al., 'The Mediator Role of Feelings of Guilt in the Process of Burnout and Psychosomatic Disorders: A cross-cultural study', *Front. Psychol.*, 12 (28 December, 2021), https://doi.org/10.3389/fpsyg.2021.751211

'Catch your critic'

Adapted from McKay, M. and Fanning, P., *Self-esteem: A proven program of cognitive techniques for assessing, improving, and maintaining your self-esteem* (New Harbinger, 2016)

'If you're not in the arena also getting your ass kicked, I'm not interested in your feedback'

YouTube, 'Brené Brown: Why Your Critics Aren't The Ones Who Count' (2013), https://youtu.be/8-JXOnFOXQk?si=pUYKuUA61VW1ouP5

Acknowledgements

To Ben – I do not know where to start in telling you how grateful I am to have you in my life. I am so lucky to be married to my best friend and my soulmate. The burnout was an awful time for both of us, and I will forever be grateful for all your support and love through that period. I cannot express in words what having you by my side has meant to me. I still have to pinch myself that you are always there cheering me on and loving me. The family we have built together is my everything. I treasure every moment with you. I love you. Thank you.

To Lyla and Artie – I have cried many tears over the months and years that I lost to burnout when you were both so little. I so deeply regret that I was not able to be the mother that you deserved back then. I have worked so hard to get better, and I have done it for you. Every day I am so happy that I am your mum. I get the absolute joy of watching you grow up to be the most incredible people. I am so very proud of you and love you both more than you will ever comprehend... but you still need to tidy your bedrooms and PUT YOUR CLOTHES AWAY!!!

To Mum, Dad and the rest of my family – you have seen me right through from being a determined teenager wanting to do nothing else but medicine, through all the blood, sweat, tears (and often other bodily fluids!), long days, nights and weekends. You know how much this career meant to me and how painful it has been to come through this period. Thank you for supporting me through this period of transition, it means so much.

To Aishah- thank you for being my business bestie, for all the 20-minute-long voice notes, and for being there through all of the ups and downs. Love you.

To Kim – where would I be without your support and a continuous feed of memes and reels! I'm so thankful for your presence in my life.

To my oldest friends who have been present for years during both the good times and the not so good! Bendy, Laura, James, Chris and Gary, thank you for being there and for always being happy to pick up where we left off.

To everyone that has offered their professional advice, support and guidance on my post-burnout career journey, thank you! There are far too many of you to mention. But please know that every single meeting, message, email, DM and voice note has helped!

To my contributors – huge thanks to Leah, Kirsty and Dan for trusting me with your stories, and for your courage in sharing them so openly. I truly hope that you are all able to find peace and contentment after your burnouts. Zoe, thank you for sharing your lived experience with ADHD, and your professional experience as a clinician – your insights were invaluable.

To Holly – I couldn't write the Acknowledgement section without mentioning you! I am so incredibly grateful that you offered me the opportunity to write this book. I have had the best experience with you being my editor, I honestly couldn't have asked for better. Thank you so much for all of your advice and guidance! I would also like to acknowledge the wider team at Bloomsbury, and to thank every single person that has worked on this book, whether we've had direct contact or not – I've had the best experience.

To the medical team that supported me through my burnout – I honestly do not know where I would be had I not received support through Practitioner Health during my burnout. You offered me support and a safe space when I was at my most vulnerable, and the course of therapy I had has not only helped me to get over my burnout, but it's also given me skills and strategies that have kept me well since. I am eternally grateful – thank you.

To the NHS Clinical Entrepreneur Team – it is not an exaggeration to say that getting a place on this programme changed my life. Thank you to Tony for creating and heading the programme, all of the support and admin team, Polly, Emily, Lucy, and everyone else. Thank you, Tamsin, for being my biggest cheerleader and for all the emotional support you have given me whilst I have been on the programme (as you said, one day this will all make an incredible success story!). Pravina, thank you for being my mentor and an absolutely invaluable source of advice and direction. But the biggest thanks goes to my fellow entrepreneurs for being the best cheerleaders ever. You all know who you are, there are too many of you to mention, but please know I am eternally grateful for your support.

To all of my followers on social media, a huge THANK YOU because ultimately you made this book possible! When I started sharing my journey with burnout on social media, I did so because I felt desperately lonely and isolated, and I couldn't believe that I was the only person that felt this way. I had no idea that what I was sharing would resonate with so many people, let alone build such an amazing community around me. If you hadn't supported my posts, I wouldn't have carried on talking about my experiences, and I wouldn't have ended up writing this book. You made this possible.

Index